Bright Side oτ the Road

Bright Side
of the
Road

A Spiritual Journey
Through Breast Cancer

Bright blessings,
Anne Marie Bennett

ANNE MARIE BENNETT

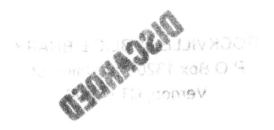

Author's Note: This book is a memoir. The events included here all happened to me and are recounted as I remember them. Some incidents have been woven together for sake of time and space, and some names have been changed. Any errors are my own.

ISBN# 1442173882

Book & cover design by Joanna Powell Colbert
www.gaiandesign.com
Cover art- *Create Your Own Reality*, by Melissa Harris
www.melissaharris.com
Author photograph by Stephanie Pacheco

Published by
KALEIDOSOUL MEDIA
PO Box 745
Beverly MA 01915
www.kaleidosoul.com

Dedication

For every woman whose journey is interrupted
by a breast cancer diagnosis:

May you realize that the road doesn't end.
May you be given the courage to embrace your journey's
twists and turns.
May you find the way to your own
bright side of the road.

Table of Contents

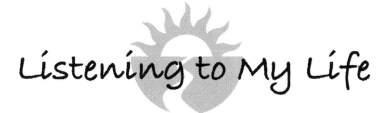

Listening to My Life

*Listen to your life. See it for the fathomless mystery that it is,
in the boredom and pain of it, no less than in the excitement and gladness:
touch, taste, smell your way to the holy and hidden heart of it, for in the last
analysis, all moments are key moments, and life itself is grace.*
— Frederick Buechner

This book is about my ten-month journey with breast cancer, beginning in December of 2001. I started out writing only about the breast cancer part: the do-over mammogram, the biopsy, the diagnosis, the surgeries, the chemotherapy, the radiation treatments, and the after-effects of all of this. But I soon realized that my breast cancer journey was in part defined by the larger story of my life's path. With predictably-perfect 20/20 hindsight, I can now see how everything that came before my breast cancer diagnosis was my own personal and perfect preparation. As ill-equipped and bewildered as I felt when I first stumbled out onto the highway of hospitals and doctors and drugs, my life prior to this journey was the only map, the only set of directions that I had… and I can see now that it was all I needed.

With this in mind, I have spent some time "listening to my life" as it was before breast cancer interrupted it. I share it with you here as a way to give background and image to the person you will meet (me!) at the beginning of Chapter 1.

Please consider this Introduction a reminder to listen to your own life... to accept your life exactly as it is, to forgive yourself for any boredom and pain within it, to celebrate the mystery of every moment of it, to deeply root yourself in the "holy and hidden heart of it," and to keep in the foreground of your beautiful mind that your life is also framed and woven with grace.

My life's journey began on May 20, 1956. I had a good childhood, as childhoods go, being born into a family of two loving parents and two older brothers who wanted me and were always there for me. We weren't wealthy, but we weren't poor either. The memories of my New England girlhood are not of vacations in shiny hotels or birthday parties at fancy restaurants. My memories are of family trips to local attractions, hikes in the nearby woods, vacations in a small cottage on the Connecticut shore, paper bag dramatics at Girl Scout camp, and laughter around the family dinner table on birthdays, Thanksgiving and Christmas.

From my father I learned creativity, humor, and unconditional love. He was artistic and often drew little cartoons for me, helped me with school projects that required some kind of art, and was very creative when it came to gift giving. He often wrote poems and sent clues in the mail weeks ahead of a special gift, to spark anticipation. In my teens, he was usually the buffer between my mother and me, smoothing and soothing our relationship, assuaging my teenage angst with his calm and steady presence.

From my mother I learned creativity, empathy, and the true pleasure of giving to others. When I was nine, she volunteered to be our troop's Girl Scout Leader, ensuring that Girl Scouting was available to me, and because of this she was able to give me leadership and social opportunities that I would not have had otherwise. My natural tendency, as a child and even now, is that of solitude. Left alone to my own devices, I would probably have spent every free waking moment in my room with the door shut, reading a book or writing a story, daydreaming, listening to records. I believe that she saw this and tried to balance my solitary tendencies with the exact opposite. I still loved those hours of reading and writing and dreaming, but my mother saw to it that my teenage years were balanced with friends, volunteering, and community action.

My brothers, being quite a bit older than me (Joe by ten years and John by six), were not around much during my growing up years. By the time I was eight years old, Joe had left for Boston University and John was already in high school. It was a wide gap, but wide only in years, not in love. In high school, I was astonished to hear stories of friends whose big brothers had tormented and teased them while growing up. I experienced none of that because of the difference in our ages.

When I was 15, Joe and his new wife Karen took me to see the musical *Man of La Mancha* at the University of Connecticut. This was my first introduction to live theatre, and it was love at first sight. They encouraged this new passion in me by taking me to many more musicals and plays during my teenage years, and I will always be grateful to them for this.

I also have dear, sweet memories of John who spent time with me playing Battleship and Radio Station, and just goofing around. When I was eleven and he was seventeen, he would take study breaks and come into my room late at night (when I was supposed to be sleeping) to tell me stories, or listen to my stories. He answered my questions about sex and boys and love as best he could, and nurtured me with just the right amount of attention and affection during my preteen years when I was typically reluctant to accept them from my parents. We were unusually close (I see now) for siblings with a six year age difference. He personified the phrase "big brother" to me in a way that still brings a smile and deep warmth to my soul when I think of it.

The sweetness of my youth was marred only by the consequences of my mother's own difficult childhood. Her father and grandfather were alcoholics, but I was well into my thirties before I realized the significance of this. Even though my mother never touched a drop of liquor herself, she was deeply and perpetually affected by the disease of alcoholism.

I am still working on the issue of forgiving my grandfather and great-grandfather for the emotional and physical abuse they inflicted on my mother when she was a child. The stories that she told me are laden with shame and humiliation, and they wreak havoc in my heart. She never spoke of happy childhood memories, and that in itself tells me much about the burden of sorrow that her own life contained.

After my dad died in 1993 at the age of 72, she lived alone for eleven years until her own death while I was writing this book. A few months before she died, I told her that I saw her as a strong woman with many gifts and that I greatly admired her. Her eyes filled with tears and she reached for my hand. It occurred to me then that no one in the eight decades of her life had ever told her that. I smiled through my own tears and held her hand tightly. It felt incredibly good to be able to give her this gift.

During my adolescence I was busy studying, hanging out with friends, reading, playing my guitar, singing in the chorus, babysitting, assisting a Brownie troop, working part time at the library, and filling innumerable notebooks with handwritten pages of stories and novels.

My spiritual life was beginning at this time also. My family was Catholic and when I was little, we went to church every Sunday. By my teen years, I was the only one going to church. My father claimed claustrophobia and my mother claimed her bad knees as their excuses but I couldn't help wondering if their aversion to church was something deeper than this. Either way, I faithfully went to Mass every Saturday night on my own. Perhaps I went simply because my parents *didn't* go and this was one way of forging my independence. Or perhaps I went out of a deeper need for community, a stronger sense of faith.

When we were sixteen, my best friend Theresa went on a youth retreat and came back aglow with the fire of having "accepted Jesus Christ as her Lord and Saviour." I caught the flame, so to speak, and gave my own life to Jesus after listening to her story. I began studying the Bible on my own, making prayer lists, and seriously considering all things of God. I was fortunate because my mother's best friend (whom I called "Auntie Hazel") lived in the apartment upstairs from us. She was Episcopalian and had many, many years of experience in the practice of her faith, and she was not shy about sharing it with me. Now and then she would take me aside, talk to me about her experiences in prayer, loan me books, pray with me. She also was a much-needed buffer between my mother and me during those adolescent years.

My parents expected me to go to college and I didn't question this. I wanted this experience, craved it even, looked forward to being away from home. When I questioned myself about what I wanted to do with my life, the answer that always arose was *I want to be a writer.* But I also knew that writing didn't necessarily provide a steady income, so I decided to be a teacher, thus indulging one of my secondary passions- a deep love and respect for children.

College in New Haven was at first lonely and frightening even though I was only an hour away from home. I felt like a goldfish plucked out of her tiny bowl and dropped into the ocean. But in time I began to experience a satisfying equilibrium, realizing that I was able to swim, that I wouldn't drown. The freedom was undeniably wonderful, and even more wonderful as I began to make friends and take steps towards creating my own life. I was intent on becoming a teacher; all of my energies were focused on this goal. Several of my friends were planning to get married and have children right away, but I didn't want any part of that. I wanted my own life; I wanted to travel and live on my own a while before settling down. I experienced one serious relationship but mostly dated casually, sporadically.

I attended Bible Studies and prayer groups throughout college, attended Christian retreats, studied hard and joined several campus organizations including Glee Club, Student National Education Association, and the Yearbook Committee. Most of my friends at that time were what we then called "born again Christians." Faith was simple. Life was fun. Love was easy.

I graduated Magna Cum Laude in May of 1978. Teaching jobs in Connecticut at that time were scarce, but I had meant it when I said that I would go anywhere if they'd let me have my own classroom. At the end of that summer I was hired to teach second grade in a rural farming community in Virginia, six hundred miles from everything and everyone I knew (and thirty miles away from the nearest mall!). Some of my friends thought I was crazy, but I didn't think twice. Many people told me I was courageous but I never saw it that way. It was difficult, packing up my black and white Dodge Dart Swinger and driving away, leaving both of my parents weeping silently on the sidewalk in front of our house. This was the first time I'd seen my father cry and it made a lasting impression on me. I wept all the way to New Jersey.

I lived and taught in Amelia for six years, and was very happy there. I was finally living my own life: teaching, making friends, taking summer vacations, and going home every year for Christmas. I officially joined the Episcopal Church my first year there and became part of the tiny family at Christ Church. I made friends with Gail, a fourth grade teacher and we shared an apartment. We joined an interdenominational Bible Study and Prayer Group that had a big impact on my life. The couples and individuals in this group were my family while I was living in Virginia.

After four years, Gail moved to Fredericksburg so I had the apartment to myself. While I was enjoying the solitude, I found myself quite lonely. This is when Patrick entered my life. He was hired by the local high school to teach history and coach basketball. I met him at a county-wide faculty meeting in September and immediately felt sorry for him, being the new Yankee in town (he was from Pennsylvania). He had also moved there not knowing anyone and I empathized completely.

Patrick and I became friends quickly. In spite of his passion for basketball, golf and baseball, we did have several things in common, including a love of good books and movies, funny stories, Mexican food, dancing, and music from the sixties. I let some of my walls down with him, and before I knew what was happening, I was crazy in love with him. This might have been a good thing except for the fact of his alcoholism which I was blissfully in denial of until it was too late.

A year later I was feeling burned-out from six years of teaching, and decided that I'd had enough of living so far away from my family. My brothers were both creating families of their own and I was longing to get to know my nieces and nephews. I moved to Boston and took a job with an educational consulting company. There were many schools in eastern Massachusetts that had just purchased our learning software and I was the link between the school and the corporate offices. I opened an office, hired staff, and joined corporate America in a way that was still being true to my spirit. I was working with children, teachers and administrators. I felt that I was making a difference in education in a way that I wasn't able to as a teacher.

As for Patrick, the alcoholism was taking over his life. He had been fired from his teaching job and gone back to Pennsylvania. Our relationship lasted off and on for four more years. I still deeply loved him, even though I knew I was putting my life on hold for someone who couldn't fully love me in return.

Eventually (thanks to my brother John) I found my way to Al-Anon, and my life changed immeasurably. For the first time since leaving Virginia, I found myself in a supportive, loving community where I wasn't afraid or ashamed to ask for help. These people, who loved the alcoholics in their lives as much as I loved Patrick, helped me to find my way back to my faith in a power greater than myself. Eventually I developed enough inner strength to end the relationship with Patrick.

This reconnection to my faith affected my life profoundly. I felt stirrings within to return to the Church, so after I moved to Salem (one year in Boston was enough for me!), I joined St. Peter's Episcopal Church and immediately felt at home. Because this was a much larger parish than my previous church in Virginia, I was able to let myself be ministered to instead of feeling like I had to join committees and "do" things. My first months there were spent drinking in the liturgy, the music, the rector's intuitive wisdom, and the presence of the Spirit that I had chosen to ignore for so long. I asked Randy, the rector, for spiritual direction after he mentioned the Twelve Steps in one of his sermons. His presence in my life was one of brother, friend, and spiritual guide. He also introduced me to the practice of meditation and yoga through his weekly classes in the parish hall.

With Patrick gone, I needed a home base, and that sense of family came from St. Peter's. I joined the Prayer Group, wrote the monthly newsletter, became a Lay Eucharistic Minister, and assisted my friend Lori with our production of *Godspell*. These were some of the happiest years of my life. I knew who I was and felt like I was in exactly the right place, doing exactly the right thing.

I was writing again in my spare time which wasn't much, but it was a start. Several of my essays and articles were published in the local paper and several Christian magazines. A children's novel began nudging me also and so I wrote *My Other Dad* which I co-published with a small press in Tennessee. I began several novels and short stories but had little time or energy to focus on bringing these projects to completion.

My life was full. I was content and happy.

But I was also lonely. At thirty-five years old, my entire social life revolved around the church. In a brave effort to bolster my social life, I placed a short personals ad in the local paper:

> *The road less traveled is my path. Loving, attractive, SWF, 35, with passion for water, words, children, laughter, altars, music and theatre. Seeks creative, compassionate, fun companion for the journey. Will you join me?*

My social life did increase, almost immediately. I met quite a few nice guys, went to concerts, out to dinner, for walks on the beach. All nice guys, but I didn't really "click" with any of them.

Enter: Jeff Bennett, Bachelor #7. He was a controller for a financial company, separated, and living the next town over from me. We talked on the phone a few times and I had an immediate sense of connection with him. We made each other laugh, and I was struck with how he talked about his children who now lived with him. We met for dinner and as soon as I shook his hand, I felt like I'd come home. It went much deeper than physical attraction, although that was a big part of it. It was like I'd known him all my life. After three dates, I simply *knew* that he was the man I wanted to be with for the rest of my life.

In what seemed like an insane move to our family and friends, I moved in with him and his children, Amanda (10) and Jeffrey (7) two months later. His youngest daughter, Merri (5), still lived with their mother an hour away from us. Moving into this love, this family, felt absolutely right and I felt no qualms about doing it so quickly. The kids were wary at first but we soon became a stepfamily of sorts, and I fell in love with them as well as their father. After six months together, I was totally stressed with trying to balance career and family, so I left my consulting career behind, and went forward with Jeff and the kids.

In spite of the challenges, struggles, and growing pains of steering a stepfamily through uncharted waters, our love was growing and strengthening. Jeff and I managed to get away now and then for a romantic weekend, spending precious time on our own relationship. During these years I worked as a substitute teacher, a bookseller, and a computer teacher.

I left St. Peter's in Salem and we joined St. Peter's in Beverly as a family. We were married there in 1995. Jeff and I built a house in North Beverly that same year. Merri was still living with her mother but the divorce agreement gave us the blessing to have her with us every other weekend. These visits were welcome breaths of fresh air and sunshine as Merri was always an easygoing presence and a joy to have around.

Right after we were married, I started working part time in the Box Office of the North Shore Music Theatre, a large regional theatre in Beverly. I wanted to focus again on my writing and thought this would be the perfect opportunity to earn some money to pay the bills but still give me a good chunk of time each week to write. It *was* a good opportunity, but the next year, I was offered a fulltime position at the theatre and I took it even though it meant giving up my writing time. I chose to do this because the extra income was welcome, the environment was creative, and the extra hours kept me away from home during the turbulent times of the kids' adolescence.

When Amanda was 18, she joined the Air Force. Some things changed at the theatre, and suddenly I was not only a fulltime employee, but Assistant Box Office Manager as well. Jeffrey was dealing with his own issues, supported by Jeff's persistent unconditional love. Merri was still living with her mother and we saw her every other weekend.

Around this time I was shopping for a Mother's Day gift at a rubber stamp store at the mall. My mom was an avid rubber stamp artist. She had invited me to stamp with her on many occasions but I had always declined, thinking that there was no way *I* could create such beautiful pieces of art. As I was looking for a gift for her, I saw a note card with a beautiful sparkling butterfly on it. Curious, I asked the cashier how it was made. She pulled out a rubber stamp, embossing ink, powder and heat gun.. and showed me right there in a matter of seconds! I was immediately hooked, and ended up buying several "gifts" for myself that day, as well as my mother. This began an exciting time of creativity and joy for me as I started to explore rubber stamp art and collage with a passion I hadn't known was inside of me.

Also, up until this time I had been very active at St. Peter's in Beverly but was feeling burned-out from committee meetings and tension between certain parishioners. In the summer of 1999, I decided to take a short time off from my responsibilities there, to give myself some space and distance from all of it. We had joined that church as a family and now that our family was going off in separate directions, I wondered if it was time for me to find a church of my own, or perhaps a church for Jeff and I to join together.

Well, there you have it. A relief map (so to speak) of my life's journey before breast cancer landed in front of me like an avalanche plummeting from a nearby mountain. I have tried to be honest. To layer in the hurts along with the joys and the losses along with the blessings. I want you to have a feel for what was going on in my life before I was diagnosed. I want you to feel like you know me, at least a little bit. And most of all, I want you to trust me enough to guide you on your own journey, wherever that may be taking you.

Every woman's path is unique, both prior to her diagnosis and afterwards. And every woman, in some sense, is prepared for the journey simply by the tools she has acquired in her daily life up to that moment when her journey so drastically departs from the norm. For one it may be a lifetime of mothering and family; for another a focusing on career, friends and social events; for someone else it could be a solitary life of meditation and prayer, or any combination of the above.

We usually don't know it until life requires it of us, and it doesn't matter where our path has taken us. At any given moment we are gathering into ourselves all of the courage, strength, and wisdom that we need for the journey ahead. Come, step out onto the Bright Side of the Road with me. We will make this journey together.

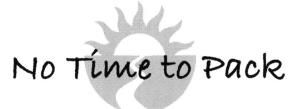

CHAPTER ONE

No Time to Pack

Just because we cannot see clearly the end of the road,
that is no reason for not setting out on the essential journey.
--- John F. Kennedy

Tuesday November 27

There's a message waiting for me from the nurse at our doctor's office when I get home tonight. Call her as soon as possible. It's urgent. I wonder what it could be. Probably some missing paperwork. Maybe I forgot to sign something. I just had my yearly physical a few weeks ago and everything was fine. Wasn't it?

Wednesday November 28

It takes several minutes of an automated maze of button pushing, but I finally reach the nurse who left the message. She tells me I need to schedule another mammogram right away because the one I had a few weeks ago looks "suspicious." My heart starts pounding in my chest and I wonder if she can hear it through the phone. She tells me not to worry; it's just routine follow-up. I ask when I should do this and she tells me this afternoon would be good. This afternoon. I swallow hard and my heart beats a bit faster.

Suzanne (my boss) looks more than a little concerned. She says I should go right now even though it's extremely busy here today.

My heart is still racing as I drive the five miles to Lahey Clinic. I guess the fight or flight mechanism built into my body has been activated by this unexpected news. Still, my mind counteracts my body's fear with reassuring whispers: *It'll be okay. Lots of women have to have second mammograms. This happens all the time. There's nothing to worry about.*

The mammogram today is especially uncomfortable because I'm in the throes of PMS and my breasts are sore and tender. I wince but don't say anything. The technician is cheerful and kind in her bright patterned jacket and golden hair.

Back in the small waiting area, I sit on a blue padded chair wearing an ugly dishwater-gray hospital gown that's too small. I'm flipping through a glossy woman's magazine which is full of articles on sex, recipes for Christmas cookies, and lovely photographs of Jennifer Anniston, but none of it penetrates my bewildered brain. There are four other women in similar chairs, waiting. One of them has had breast cancer. I know this because her hair looks like it's just starting to grow back, and she's chatting with the receptionist about surgeons and chemo treatments. I try to ignore her. They say ignorance is bliss.....I just don't want to know.

One by one the four other women are given the thumbs-up-you-can-go-home-now sign from the older woman behind the counter. One by one, I watch them leave. I close the magazine and think of statistics. What is it, one woman in eight that ends up with breast cancer? Or is it one woman in ten? Six? I can't remember. But how many women do *I* know who have had breast cancer? Absolutely none.

The odds are not in my favor.

This realization dawns on me slowly as I lay the magazine down on the table beside me and look around at the empty waiting room. What if today, *I* am the woman who *doesn't* get the thumbs-up sign?

Sure enough, in a few minutes, the golden-haired technician comes out of another room and calls my name. I stand slowly and realize that I am freezing cold and trembling. She looks at me kindly and tells me the doctor wants to speak with me for a few minutes. I am terrified. My mouth is dry;

my chest is tight. I know the doctor doesn't want to see me so he can tell me that everything is okay. Everything was okay with those four other women and they didn't need the doctor to tell them this. They are already in their cars, driving home to their safe little worlds. I am still here. The doctor wants to speak with *me*.

I follow the technician to a different examining room and wait less than a minute for the radiologist to appear. He is an older man, tall and slender. Grandfatherly in appearance yet businesslike in manner. He invites me to sit on a metal stool with wheels, but he remains standing. I am acutely aware of how awkward this feels, how powerless I feel because he is standing and I am not. He tells me there are some tiny calcifications in my left breast, calcifications that weren't there during my last mammogram a year ago. Eighty percent of the time these turn out to be nothing, he reassures me. But he wants me to make an appointment with a breast surgeon. Today if possible. The surgeon will decide if I need a biopsy.

I am speechless. Should I say something, ask some questions? I simply can't. My mind is spinning too fast to think clearly.

The technician comes back and I walk with her down the brightly lit corridor to the wing of surgeons' offices. I wonder if this is what an out-of-body experience feels like. She is chatting brightly about the weather and her Thanksgiving holiday while I am biting my lip and trying not to cry.

She leaves me with the receptionist and I pull out a piece of gum, chewing on it furiously, hoping this will make it impossible for me to break into tears. The receptionist is kind and soft-spoken, her eyes behind jeweled eyeglasses darting between me and her omniscient computer screen. She schedules the appointment for the day after tomorrow, hands me a prim white reminder card with the date and time neatly written in. Good Lord, does she really think I might *forget*?

When I get back to the office, I need to talk with my husband Jeff but don't think I can call him without crying. I email him instead and he replies immediately: *Whatever happens, we'll get through it together. I love you.* I read these words and can physically feel the love behind them. I am so grateful for this man. He has said just the right thing and my heart is eased.

After I've had sufficient time to absorb some of this, I knock on Suzanne's door and tell her a little of what has just happened, and that I will be late on Friday morning. She tells me not to worry about it, that it's more important to take care of this right away. Again, gratitude floods my heart. She too has said the right thing and this eases my worried mind.

Friday November 30

I'm sitting on a hard metal examining table in a tiny white room. The waxy paper beneath me crackles as I cross my legs. There is nothing on the walls here except a large poster advertising pain medication. There are happy and sad faces on a scale from 1 – 10 with the suggestion that I rate my current physical pain using these numbers. I wonder if anyone will ask me to rate my current *emotional* distress (surely a number much higher than 10) using those faces. Probably not.

There is a gentle knock on the sliding door, and then my surgeon enters the room. I've told myself that I will trust my intuition: if I don't like him, I will find someone else. But intuition immediately informs me that he is good, safe, kind. He's a little shorter than me, with short brown curly hair and small silver glasses. I am struck with the warmth of his smile as he reaches out to shake my hand and introduces himself as Dr. Karp.

Then he perches on the nearby desk and asks me to tell him how I'm feeling and why I'm here today.

Why am I here?

Did I hear him correctly? Is this a test question, to see how intelligent, how coherent I am? Does any woman walk into an appointment with a breast surgeon and *not* know why she's there? I think of saying *I was just in the neighborhood and thought I'd drop in to see what a breast surgeon does for a living*, but decide against it. What if he can't take a joke?

I tell him why I'm here. He nods thoughtfully as he listens, then has me lie down and open the gown so he can examine me. His hands are gentle. He helps me sit up and tells me to place my hands on his shoulders while he continues the examination. I like the feeling that this gives me, the feeling that I'm leaning on him, being supported by his knowledge, experience, wisdom.

While he examines my breasts, he asks me where I work and I tell him about the Music Theatre. He says it sounds interesting and I ask him if he's ever been to one of our shows. It seems that he's just moved to Massachusetts and hasn't had a chance to explore yet. We talk some more about the weather and then move on to life in the Boston area. I would like to continue this small talk indefinitely because it is enabling my denial of the truth which is that I'm sitting half naked in front of a surgeon who is examining my breasts for possible cancer.

Dr. Karp helps me adjust my gown and leans back again on the desk after washing his hands. Apparently the small talk is over for the day. I notice his Lahey nametag while I'm waiting. Dr. Stephen Karp. Good, I think. I've always liked the name Stephen.

He tells me that he didn't feel anything in my breasts. I ask if that's good or not, and I'm sure he can hear the vulnerability in my voice. He says that just because he didn't feel anything doesn't mean there's nothing there. Eighty percent of the time the calcifications mean nothing. He says that if he were a betting man, he'd wager good money that everything is okay. We look at the mammogram film and he points out the tiny white chalklike points of the calcifications.

Then he tells me he wants me to have a "stereotactic core biopsy." The harsh sterile sound of these words illuminate me with fear.

I get dressed and join him in the hallway. I ask if the biopsy will hurt and he tells me that most of his patients say it's no more annoying than a trip to the dentist but that a few women have described it as painful. I'm grateful for his honesty, and also for the fact that he didn't declare it painful or not painful as if he'd experienced the biopsy himself, but referred to his patients' descriptions of it instead.

Dr. Karp asks one of the nurses to go over the biopsy procedure with me and to schedule it within the week. Then he shakes my hand firmly and walks away. The nurse leads me to another tiny room. She hands me a booklet and tells me exactly what the procedure will entail. We schedule the biopsy for a week from today.

I leave the doctor's office sure of only one thing. I am no longer frightened. Dr. Karp's confidence and authoritative yet warm manner have made contact with my fear, and considerably diminished it for the time being.

Sunday December 2

The fear, better described as terror, comes back to me in waves. After all, women do die from breast cancer. No one has said that I *have* breast cancer, of course, but what if I do? What then? Will the treatments make me sick? What if it spreads? Will they have to remove my breasts? What if I die? The thoughts go whirling on and on, not only in my mind, but my heart and soul.

Tonight when I climb into bed, I give in to the fear and begin to weep uncontrollably. Jeff lies beside me, holding me tightly, letting me cry. I vaguely wonder if I should be handling this better, if I should be stronger, less afraid, more confident. But I made a promise to myself a few days ago: to cry when I need to cry. I know that inner strength doesn't really have anything to do with how many tears fall from a woman's eyes. I'm telling myself this while I'm crying, along with wondering what Jeff would do if I did die, speculating whether this might be the last *Christmas Carol* production I'll ever see, and asking myself what if this is the last time I'll hug my niece Allison who is coming from Atlanta this week to visit. The thoughts spin themselves like sticky webs across my mind until I remind myself to take a deep breath and stay in the moment. This moment. The only moment I have.

So I return to this moment and notice that I'm feeling a luscious, expansive, most wonderful love flowing from Jeff to me and back again, and I can't help the tears of gratitude that begin to flow. Yes, more tears… but these are born from the realization of an unexpected, undeserving grace. We lie together quietly for a while after my tears subside before I open myself to him. Our lovemaking is slow and sweet, and I cry some more with him inside me, treasuring our love. Have I ever treasured it this much before?

Afterwards, Jeff snores his way into sleep and I embrace him from behind. The covers are off, the windows are open a little letting in an unseasonably warm breeze. I'm filled with a deep, quiet, satisfied peace. And instead of crying with the pain of what it would be like to lose this man, this peace, this life… I am suddenly and fiercely certain of just one thing. NOTHING is going to take this away from me because I am going to fight to stay alive. If there is cancer inside of me, I'm going to fight it and I'm going to win.

I see now what I didn't see a few days ago when fear was taking control. I have a choice. And this is my choice: to claim my life, to fight for it, to do what needs to be done.

The peace within me deepens, spreads, and settles until it is all that I feel. Tonight in our bedroom with the windows open and the surprise of an April breeze blowing in December, I feel as though I've been touched by

God, or an angel, or maybe even my father who died eight years ago but still hovers nearby to comfort me. Whoever or Whatever it is, there is definitely Spirit here tonight.

I'm reminded of a quotation by medieval mystic Julian of Norwich, a passage that I was drawn to many years ago. It now comes to the forefront of my consciousness with amazing clarity. *And all shall be well and all shall be well, and all manner of thing shall be well.* I repeat this over and over in my mind. The more I say it, the more true it seems.

Tuesday December 4

I call my friend JoAnn and tell her about the biopsy, ask for her prayers. It feels good to talk about it with someone besides Jeff. The whole thing now seems a little less surreal.

I send out some emails to a few friends and my brother John, asking them to pray me through the biopsy on Friday. I feel good knowing that I have done this one thing, for it is the only thing I can do really, to prepare for it.

I'm still scared, though. So much is unknown. I'm afraid of the pain I might feel on Friday. Afraid of crying in front of strangers, of having people feel sorry for me. I have placed the words from Julian of Norwich everywhere as a reminder to me, a touchstone. They are computer-generated on little pieces of colored paper and now I see them everywhere I go: the bathroom mirror, the computer monitor at work and at home, the refrigerator, my dresser, the desk in my Quiet Room, the dashboard of my car.

And all shall be well and all shall be well, and all manner of thing shall be well.

The words become a prayer that soothes and comforts me. It is so hard not to let the *what if* mantra overpower this internal prayer. It is difficult to stay in the present moment when I am full of wishing that the whole thing was over.

Friday December 7

Jeff is driving me to the Lahey Clinic in Burlington for the biopsy. It's fifteen minutes further down the highway from Lahey Peabody and we've left early because of the traffic. He navigates well, listening to his favorite talk radio station. Every once in a while he reaches over and holds my hand. I sit on the passenger side with the latest issue of *Real Simple* magazine in my lap, hoping to distract myself from the thought of what lies ahead.

I understand from my talk with the nurse that I'm going to be lying face down on a raised table with my breast dangling through a hole, that the doctor will numb the breast and then pull out some sample cells from the area in question. The whole procedure will take a few hours and then I'll need to go home and rest. Even though I know all of this, I'm still fearful. The unknown lurks ahead of me and I want to run in the other direction. I don't know the people who'll be performing the biopsy, I don't know what the room looks like, or how I'll respond. What if I am one of the women who find it extremely painful? Dr. Karp's calm, reassuring manner seems far behind me. I can't even remember what he looks like.

As I flip through the magazine, I find myself stopping at an article entitled *How to Pray* by Lindsey Crittenden, and am struck with the perfect timing of this. It's been a long time since I actually prayed, and if ever there was a time for me to begin again, this is it. I read it carefully, grateful for the diversion. A woman priest suggests a simple prayer: *God, you are here. God, I am here.* These words are simple, yet I can feel their power as I read them, murmur them aloud, assimilate them into my body and soul. I can still feel the fear but now I know I can walk through it to the other side because I know I'm not alone. I decide to use this new prayer when I'm lying on the table, and I know that everything will be all right.

At the hospital, I follow a nurse through a maze of identical corridors. She is calm but chatty in a professionally-gauged effort to divert my attention. I listen to her but find it difficult to talk. My throat is dry and tight; my heart is beating faster than usual. She leads me to a large room with comfortable teal sofas, and I comment about how this is my favorite color. As we sit down she tells me her name is Marion, then introduces me to another nurse, Pat.

They chat about their upcoming department Christmas party until the door opens and a woman about my age walks in. She's tall and slender with short black curly hair sprinkled with wisps of gray. I like her immediately. She introduces herself as Dr. Diedrich, then warmly shakes my hand. The first thing she tells me is that the procedure is going to be completely painless. She says firmly that no patient of hers has ever felt any pain, and that I'm not going to either. I totally believe her.

I'm completely amazed that these are her first words to me. In a matter of seconds, she has taken the prime factor of my fear and completely destroyed it. For the first time this morning, I feel safe, relieved, grateful. Let the biopsy begin.

I use my new prayer while lying on the table, but not as often as I expected. The three women are including me in their humorous, effortless chatter and I find it a pleasant diversion. It's like they've made a secret pact not to let me drown in my own toxic thoughts.

Dr. Diedrich is right; I feel no pain at any time. She numbs my breast, does the biopsy, then has to start all over again to get another sample. All the while, Marion bustles around me, checking the computer screen, adjusting the table, assisting the doctor. Pat stays by my right side, talking quietly to me, asking about the theatre, telling me about her dog, chatting about the country music in the background. All the while she is rubbing my back or stroking my arm, occasionally asking me how I'm doing. Now and then I laugh out loud and Dr. Diedrich scolds them for making me laugh because my breast is jiggling. Of course, this only makes me laugh harder.

Unbelievable. I am laughing. Laughing as I lie here on this table while a radiologist takes samples of my breast tissue to see if I have cancer. Am I in denial again, or am I simply being in the moment? I realize it doesn't matter. It's getting me through a difficult morning, and this is what counts.

And does it matter that I'm not praying like I thought I would be? I think not. There are many people praying for me right now, and I'm feeling the effects of this already.

God, you are here.
God, I am here.

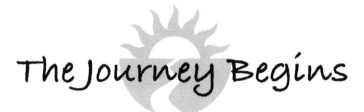

CHAPTER TWO

The Journey Begins

Things have changed here since yesterday.

— *Waiting for Godot, by Samuel Beckett*

Tuesday December 11

It's been four days since the biopsy and I'm deeply anxious to hear the results. I'm hoping against hope (now I know what this expression *really* means) that the news is good, but I'm not sure that it's going to be. My intuition, which I have learned to trust over the years, is telling me that the journey has only just begun. At 9 a.m., I call Dr. Karp's office and the secretary takes my message. She will ask him to call me.

It's busy at the Box Office but I'm finding it hard to focus on phone calls or paperwork. I call Dr. Karp's office again at 3:00. This time I tell the secretary I'm awaiting biopsy results and could she please see if they're in yet. She puts me on hold. I wait. The music playing in the background is soft and soothing, the exact opposite of my interior landscape, yet it does nothing to assuage my erratic heartbeat. Now the secretary is back on the line.

She tells me there's something wrong with her computer so she can't read the results. She reassures me that Dr. Karp will call me later.

As I hang up the phone, I'm certain there is nothing wrong with her computer. I'm thinking that if it was good news, she would have told me the results, or asked me to call back in a little while when the computer was fixed. But she didn't do either of these things. She told me the doctor would call me, and that sounds like bad news to me.

My heart beats louder the rest of the afternoon. I'm sure everyone I work with can hear it but they go about their business like it's an ordinary day. My mouth feels like it's stuffed with cotton balls and I'm having a hard time concentrating. Finally at 5:30 my phone rings and it's Dr. Karp. He tells me he's calling from the cell phone in his car and asks if that's all right. I'm strangely touched by this small courtesy, but what difference could it possibly make? He could be calling from the moon, just as long as he tells me what's happening inside my body. Now. Just tell me *now*. When I tell him that I don't mind, he doesn't waste any time (or my fear) with small talk.

There are cancerous cells in my biopsy sample.

My inner chatter, my breath, my whole world comes to a screeching halt. Cancerous cells in my body. *My* body. How can this possibly be? What can it possibly mean? My mind is spinning out of control, but the good doctor is still talking. I hear his voice but it is only a whir of noise inside the telephone. Nothing penetrates my mind right now except the C word. Cancer.

I somehow focus long enough to hear him say that he knows I'm probably upset because he's just told me I have cancer, but he wants me to remember that all cancer detected in a mammogram is very, very treatable. He wants me to remember this. I try to hold onto the words and find that *they* are hanging onto *me* instead. I ask him what he means by "treatable" and it's like I'm on the other side of the room watching myself over there at my desk. My voice sounds dry and shaky. I see myself grab a pen and a ticket envelope in an attempt to write down every word he says. I know that what he's saying is important, but my hand is trembling and my mind feels totally disconnected from my body. This makes writing difficult, to say the least.

Dr. Karp mentions surgery, chemotherapy treatments, radiation and tamoxifen. I can't help thinking how blasé he sounds while he is telling me how treatable my cancer is. Strangely, this infuriates and reassures me at the same time. He must diagnose hundreds of women each year. He knows which reports indicate grave danger and which ones don't. He definitely doesn't sound worried and I decide right now that this is a good thing. He reassures me that he'll go over everything in more detail with me on Friday at my next appointment.

In a moment our connection is gone and he is traveling down Route 128, probably on his way home to his family and a nice warm dinner. I'm sitting at my desk, staring at the black office phone, wondering exactly what I'm on *my* way to.

I'm acutely aware that my life as I know it is now over. Somewhere in the back of my mind it occurs to me that this might not be such a bad thing, but I leave that thought there, in the back of my mind, for closer inspection at another time.

When I was young, I loved it when my dad would grab me by the hands and spin me round and round in circles. Then, back on solid earth again, the world would still be spinning and I wouldn't quite know which way to go. That was fun then, all those years ago- a game, a delight. But it's not amusing now.

Dazed and disoriented, I manage to steer myself through the lobby to the ladies room where I sit on the floor of the handicapped stall and cry quietly into my hands. I'm wondering why Dr. Karp didn't say *You Have Cancer* instead of *There Were Cancerous Cells In Your Biopsy.* Because no matter how it's phrased, it all boils down to the fact that I have cancer.

I. Have. Cancer.

I can say these words in my head, but the brutal fact of it is still beyond my grasp.

Several minutes pass before it occurs to me that I have to go back to work. I dry my eyes with toilet paper, and somehow manage to go back to my desk and get some more work done. I know I could leave and everyone would understand, but I don't want to leave yet. I'm not quite ready to walk out of this brightly lit room that's buzzing with good and familiar energy. I want to sit here a bit longer and get my bearings before venturing out into the cold dark night. Or maybe I'm thinking that if I just stay still, just sit here at my desk, making these phone calls, doing this paperwork, that nothing will change, that I won't have to deal with any of this.

After half an hour, my coworker John leans over and asks if I'm okay. We've worked together for three years now and his desk is next to mine. I've always felt a kinship with him. I tell him what my doctor just told me and find myself using the same words: cancerous cells in my biopsy sample. To me, this sounds much milder than saying outright that I have cancer, but John's gentle expression of concern turns to outright dismay. Since before the biopsy, he's been telling me that I will be all right and I longed to believe him. Now he is looking at me with genuine fear and worry written all over his handsome young face.

I'm surprised to find myself reassuring him that I'm all right. There's a deadly disease inside of me, but for some reason I'm making it my job to comfort others. I grasp onto Dr. Karp's words and confidence as I tell John that what I have is treatable and if my doctor isn't worried about it, then I'm not worried about it either. He nods as he listens but looks doubtful, and we both go back to the paperwork on our desks. Perhaps I'm minimizing the reality of all of this. Perhaps I'm in active, creative denial. Perhaps this is the only way to get through these next few hours without falling apart completely.

I feel glad that John is beside me, that he has cared enough to ask what the doctor said. Glad that I have told someone, that the world did not implode when I did.

On the short drive home, I wonder how to tell Jeff about the cancer. Should I say what Dr. Karp told me, that there are "cancerous cells" in my left breast tissue? Should I just blurt out the words *I have breast cancer*? Or should I .... What? What other options are there, really? I've read thousands of self-help books and magazine articles in my life, but have never come across one entitled *How To Tell Your Husband You Have Breast Cancer*.

I know I'm going to cry. This is why I didn't call him from the theatre. The tears have been building inside of me for the last three hours and they desperately need a line of escape. I'm reminded of the story of the little boy who falls down a flight of stairs and then just sits on the bottom step, stunned by the fall, bewildered by the sudden pain. His mother runs to him and picks him up, cradling him to her. Then and only then does the little boy finally begin to cry; for in her arms it is safe to feel his pain. There in her arms is the blessed possibility of comfort.

I feel like the little boy, still sitting on the bottom step, stunned into immobility. It's not really safe to cry just yet.

Entering the house, I inhale the warmth as I close the door to the cold winter evening behind me. There's a lump in my throat the size of a ragged apple core and I can feel tears burning my eyelids. Jeff is in the bedroom, reading the paper. For a moment I envy him his ignorance. I set my purse down on the bed and blurt out the news, using the *cancerous cells* euphemism instead of the stark word *cancer*.

He comes to me, arms open for immediate embrace. I let myself be held, feeling just like the little boy who fell down the stairs. This… here… is my safety. Tears pour out of me with irrepressible momentum. Jeff strokes my back, my hair; saying over and over again that it's okay, that everything is going to be all right, that we'll get through this together.

I don't want this! I don't want this! I sob over and over into Jeff's chest. I say it so many times that it takes me back to my teaching days and the creative drama exercise where I had each student repeat the same sentence several times, each time putting the stress on a different word to see how it changes the meaning.

I don't want this.

I *don't* want this.

I don't *want* this.

I don't want *this*.

But no matter which word I stress, the meaning is the same. I feel an agonizing anger that this is happening to me and I wish with all my strength that it wasn't happening. But it is. I feel like I'm dreaming…. only I know for sure it's not a dream. The reality is, there is cancer in my body. No matter how many stars I wish on, it will remain so. I continue to cry while these thoughts spin through my mind like a dizzying, burning sandstorm.

Jeff continues to hold me. He holds me and holds me and holds me until I think I can stand on my own.

CHAPTER THREE

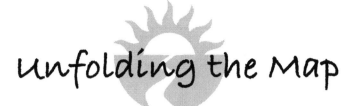

Unfolding the Map

Following the light of the sun, we left the Old World.
— Christopher Columbus

Wednesday December 12

This morning I tell my boss, Suzanne, about the biopsy results. She is so kind to me that I can feel a new batch of tears building in my throat. Somehow she manages to show just the right amount of concern and compassion. She seems to know that too much will surely push me right off the edge of this emotional cliff I'm trying to avoid, and too little would make me think she doesn't care. She tells me that her mother had breast cancer many years ago. All she had to have was several weeks of radiation treatments and now she's fine. I'm bolstered by the hope that this knowledge gives me. Could my own breast cancer treatment really be that simple?

I get through the work day in a murky inner haze. Can it really be true that I have cancer? I haven't yet been able to work up the courage to tell anyone else. I don't want my theatre family feeling sorry for me; I don't think I could bear that. The whole thing is taking up space in my mind and body, and by day's end I'm exhausted with trying to assimilate its presence into my life.

Tonight after dinner Jeff and I sit on the couch, snuggled together watching an old *Seinfeld* rerun. I love sitting next to him like this, feeling his warmth, relishing his nearness, treasuring our laughter. Yes, we are laughing, in spite of it all.

Several years ago when I was an Educational Consultant, I used to give workshops for the teachers in my district, and one of the topics I researched and presented was humor: in the classroom, in one's daily life, as medicine, as stress relief. I firmly believe in the power of laughter to heal and have decided that I'm going to incorporate funny movies and TV shows and books into what is happening to me now. This is one thing that I can do.

It seems the *only* thing at the moment, so when *Seinfeld* ends and the next show is a crime drama, I start flipping through the channels with the remote, hoping for something else that will make us laugh. Eventually I land on a public television station with a comedy about an Anglican woman priest. It's unbelievably funny and we're laughing so hard we're missing some of the lines. At the end I wait for the credits and see that it is called *The Vicar of Dibley*.

I sit on the sofa for a few moments after it's over, allowing the effects of the evening's laughter to penetrate my weary body, mind and soul. Here is something to be grateful for, in spite of the fact that I have cancer. And yes, there are going to be things that inspire gratitude, even something as simple as discovering a new television show that makes me laugh. I am thoroughly delighted with this discovery.

Thursday December 13

I still can't quite grasp the fact that I have cancer. It's beyond my belief of who I am and what my life is supposed to be like. There are cancer cells in my breast, *my* left breast. Even now as I write this, they are here, here in my body. This infuriates me. I love my breasts. The men in my life have always loved my breasts. They're mine. *Mine.* MINE!!!! I want to scream ***GET THESE DAMNED CANCER CELLS OUT OF ME. I DON'T WANT THEM IN MY BODY.***

Oh, I'm sure Dr. Karp intends to get them out. He sounded so matter-of-fact, telling me about it the other night on the phone. Okay. So he can make it all go away. But. It can come back. What if it's in other parts of my body right now and I just don't know it yet?

Have I made myself sick? Have I brought this on myself? But how? Feelings not spoken? Bitterness and resentments simmering beneath the surface? Ancient grief buried within my body? I've read some of Bernie Siegel's work over the years and I know a little bit about the mind-body connection. I always assumed that people with cancer could have avoided it somehow, but now that I have it (now that *I* have it), I can see it's not quite that simple. I'm thinking that perhaps I need a therapist. An older, wiser woman who's been through this already, someone who can take my hand and show me the way. Someone I'm not afraid to cry in front of. I'm wondering if I'm brave enough. For therapy. For breast cancer. For all that lies ahead of me now.

The hardest part so far has been saying the words out loud to someone else, and I've only told three people- John and Suzanne at work, and my husband Jeff. I decide not to tell anyone else until after my appointment with Dr. Karp tomorrow. Then I will know exactly what the treatment is before I start talking about it. Knowledge is power, or so they say. Maybe I won't even tell anyone until after Christmas. I still have time to decide.

Friday December 14

This is so bizarre! My doctor is examining my breasts while my husband sits a few feet away from us. If it were any situation other than this, it might actually be amusing. But what other situation would it be? I am distracted right back to the matter at hand.

Dr. Karp once again is gentle, thorough, kind. As I place my hands on his shoulders for the first part of the exam, I feel like he's letting me lean on him again, and this adds to my feeling of safety. I can't remember any doctor's visit in my entire life where I, the patient, was invited to touch the doctor in any way.

After he's carefully examined me, he helps me sit up and I go to the chair next to Jeff. Dr. Karp leaves the room while I put on my bra and favorite turquoise sweater which I've purposely worn today because it usually makes me feel happy, safe, peaceful. I sit down next to Jeff and hold his hand, suddenly feeling none of those things yet still grateful for the reminder that they do exist.

When Dr. Karp comes back, he sits at the little table beside us and pulls out a notebook with written information and an erasable page for him to draw on. He uses it frequently as he explains what infiltrating ductal cancer really is. I notice that he's using words we can understand, and yet I don't feel like he's talking down to us.

My own notebook is in my lap, a daily organizer covered with a beautiful dark tapestry design. I'm trying to write down everything he says. When I bought it a few weeks ago, I had visions of filling it with other things: plans for selling my collage note cards, ideas for stories to write, colorful quotes, dreams. I would never have expected to be sitting here in a doctor's office filling it with notes on the type of cancer I've been told I have.

I've always found note-taking easy, but today it's much more difficult. Perhaps because I've not heard or used many of these words before. Cancer. IDC. Precancerous cells. Lymph nodes. Lumpectomy. Sentinel node biopsy. I used to love taking French and Spanish classes in high school and college. I excelled in these classes. But this is different. The foreign language that is cancer is not a lesson I signed up for.

He's very serious, this doctor of mine. I notice this while trying to translate his words into my notebook. He is serious and he is thorough. He doesn't smile much as he's explaining my options. I find myself wishing he'd be a little more cheerful, maybe even make a few jokes. But then I think, this is my *life* he's talking about. My *body*, my *life*. What kind of jokes could he possibly make? And suddenly I'm grateful for his solemn attention, for the way he's presenting this information to us visually as well as orally.

He tells us that there are no studies that show a higher rate of recurrence if a woman with Stage 2 breast cancer has a mastectomy versus a lumpectomy. Therefore he strongly recommends a lumpectomy. I breathe a soft sigh of relief when I hear this.

With that decision out of the way, I still have two choices. I can have a sentinel node biopsy, where he will take out just the first lymph node in my left armpit. If the cancer has spread to this sentinel node, they'll have to do a second surgery and take all of the lymph nodes out (an axillary node dissection). What they find during this surgery will determine my course of treatment. OR I can have the axillary node surgery instead of the sentinel node biopsy. The only problem with having all the lymph nodes out at once is that there are all kinds of side effects from it- longer recovery time, numb armpit, possible nerve damage, maybe even lymphedema. My vocabulary continues to grow.

Jeff and I aren't saying much, just listening, trying to absorb all of this new information as if there might be an exam sometime soon. Once, when Dr. Karp is talking about survival statistics, I steal a glance at Jeff, trying to imagine what he's thinking. Is this what he signed up for when he married me? Is he wishing he hadn't married me? Is he afraid? It's hard to tell because his eyes don't meet mine as he continues to focus intently on what the doctor is saying.

After a while, Dr. Karp leans back in his chair and asks if we have any questions for him. Even though I usually have more than enough questions when learning something new, I am stunned into silence. I have no idea what I should be asking. He encourages me to get a second opinion if I want one, because he's going to be with me for the long haul and he wants me to be sure that I want him as my doctor. This surprises me. I have no idea what he means by the *long haul.*

I look at my watch. We've been in this examining room for almost ninety minutes. He hasn't looked at his watch once. As we shake his hand and get up to leave, I'm certain of only one thing. This man with the gentle hands and solemn expression is going to be my doctor, my surgeon. For however long it takes.

In the car I tell Jeff I've decided to have the sentinel node biopsy and he agrees with me, but I suspect he would agree with me no matter what I decided. He says how much he likes Dr. Karp, how he likes the fact that he seems to be about our age. As he turns on the radio, I look out the window. The sky is gray and cloudy, perfectly dismal, an amazingly accurate picture of my own interior weather.

At home, in the safety of our bedroom, I begin to cry and Jeff holds me tightly, rocking me back and forth, a motion I have always found sooth-ing. The stress of *Not Knowing* versus the stress of *Knowing* has taken its toll. I'm still congested and exhausted from a head cold, not enough sleep, and the sheer effort of trying to hold it all together. My tears are sloppy and they soak into my husband's shirt. But still he holds me. I think I could drown him with my tears, but he would hold me even then.

After a while, my tears slow down. It's almost noon. Jeff leaves for work and I sit on the edge of the bed for a while in silence, feeling numb, exhausted, wrung-out. I try to wrap my mind around this new unwelcome direction my life seems to be taking without my consent. I try to at least find a space for it, since I can't really embrace it yet. Because, no matter how much I don't want breast cancer, it is here and I'm somehow going to have to find the strength to deal with it, live with it, accept it.

I wander into Jeff's study and turn on the computer, log onto the internet and visit several bulletin boards dedicated to breast cancer patients. One of them is called the Breast Cancer Survivor's Board. I'm not sure I belong there, or even have the right to post a message on it (after all, I haven't survived anything yet, have I?), but I do anyway. I ask for advice on how to tell the people in my life that I have breast cancer. I ask for advice on how to deal with all of this spiritually. It feels incredibly good to be reaching out for help. I have the medical information I need; now I need to find some women who can show me how to manage all of this with some measure of grace and humor.

Still exhausted, but having run out of tears for now, I sit in the silence and try to decide if I should go to work for the rest of the day. This is our busiest time of year at the Box Office. I know this. But I also know that I've just been diagnosed with cancer, and that guilt can no longer be a guiding light for me as far as my work life is concerned. They've gotten along fine without me all morning. I'm quite sure they can survive the afternoon as well. But do I really want to sit at home for several more hours? Do I want to sit here on this dreary cold day and think about cancer hour after hour? I've made my decision about the surgery. What will I gain by sitting here alone until Jeff comes home? I don't have enough energy for my art, or enough focus for reading or watching a movie. The thought of sitting with my thoughts and worries whirling around inside my head for several hours makes me shudder.

Eventually I stand up, move slowly to the bathroom where I splash cold water on my face and stare at myself in the mirror for several long heart-felt moments. Then I make myself a sandwich and drive to the theatre where I find bright lights, ringing phones, abundant energy, familiar faces. I tell Suzanne that I really don't feel up to answering phones right now but I'd be happy to enter subscription renewals into the computer for the rest of the day. She says that's perfectly fine. Everyone here is glad to see me and I'm grateful for this place which feels like a second home to me, these people who feel like family. They all know I was meeting with the breast surgeon this morning, yet no one asks me what he said. I know some women would be angry about this, but I feel like they're respecting my privacy and that feels good to me right now. My emotions are still very close to the surface (now I really know what *that* expression means) and I'm afraid that if I talk about it, any of it, I will break down and cry, and I'm not ready to do that here.

A few hours later I've calmed myself with the simple repetitive task of paperwork. I feel a little more like myself again, so I knock on Suzanne's door and tell her that I will need three days off for the surgery. Once again, she is kind and sympathetic, yet I don't feel pitied. She reaffirms what I already know, telling me that the most important thing is to take care of myself, to take as many days as I need.

Later in the afternoon, as the light outside my window softens into dusk, I come to a decision. *I have breast cancer and I'm going to survive it. It's not going to kill me; it's just going to be one more interesting thing about me.*

I have no idea on God's sweet earth where this thought has come from, but I seize and embrace it, clutch it to my heart like a drowning woman would grab at an inner tube thrown to her from a rescue ship. And I decide to believe it with all of my being- body, mind and soul. Just one more interesting thing. Yes, that's exactly right. I have a passion for cats and Broadway musicals and empty notebooks. I sincerely love long walks, the ocean, and good music. I am a writer and an artist. I make beautiful collage cards. Now I can add the detail of breast cancer to that list.

I think of the numerous breast cancer survivors I've seen on the *Rosie O'Donnell Show*. I recall articles in women's magazines about breast cancer survivors. I think of the women on the web bulletin boards whose stories I read this morning. And I'm beginning to sense a glimmer of hope.

CHAPTER FOUR

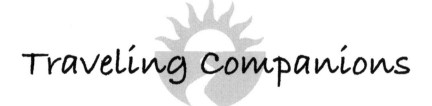

Traveling Companions

One word frees us of all the weight and pain in life. That word is love.
— Sophocles

Saturday December 15

This glimmering hope continues to grow when I go online and find dozens of responses to my post from yesterday on the Survivor's Bulletin Board. I grow the tiniest bit more encouraged with each one I read, and when I'm done, those minuscule bits of hope have added up to something more tangible. Women who've been through every conceivable stage and variety of breast cancer have written to me, welcoming me to the website. Many of them say they're sorry I have to be there but they're glad I introduced myself.

In response to my statement about how I'm not sure I belong on this board because I'm not a survivor yet, one woman reassures me that I am indeed a survivor. After all, she points out, I've survived three very difficult things already: the biopsy, the diagnosis, and the painful reality of telling a few people that I have breast cancer.

A response from a woman in Toronto also speaks deeply to my soul.

Her name is Elizabeth and she's been out of treatment for almost a year. She speaks of breast cancer as a journey, and this word whispers something vital to my soul.

I write back to her. Instinct tells me that she is a kindred spirit and that she'll be able to help me through the twists and turns that my own journey is starting to take. She replies almost immediately with more words of reassurance and hope.

I tell her I'm unsure of who to share my news with, and am even more uncertain about how to tell them. I don't know how people will react, and I don't want the added stress of worrying about their feelings while I'm telling them. She responds that she knows women who didn't tell *anybody* they had breast cancer, and women who told absolutely *everyone* they knew. She chose to be part of the latter group, and she's glad because she found wonderful blessings and support in many surprising places. However, she reminds me that the decision is mine alone to make. She also tells me not to be so worried about how others are taking the news that I forget how *I'm* taking it. She's right, of course. I need to stay focused within.

Her advice has made my decision easy. I'm going to tell everyone I know that I have cancer. I'm curious about how the people I know and love will respond to this news. I've never liked being the center of attention, but I realize that perhaps this attention, focused on me, can be a force of love and healing that will only do me good as I go forward on this journey.

I check my messages on the Survivor's Board again and am heartened by the women who've reached out to me. I feel less alone now, a little less frightened.

As I do some web searches using the phrase "breast cancer," I notice that the long computer table is dusty, covered with Jeff's papers and files. He's an accountant with quite a few clients and every one of them has an excess of necessary paperwork, all of which is cluttering up the space. I suddenly have a burning need to make this space a little bit more my own for a while. I have the feeling that I'm going to be sitting here more than usual during the coming months, so I begin to create a little altar beside the computer.

I take everything off of the table and dust it until it shines. I put Jeff's things back in their proper piles, straighten out the tangled paper clips and rubber bands, attempting to make some order from the chaos. Perhaps some of this order will find its way into my own messy soul.

I carry up the green and purple stained glass lamp from the living room, along with the vanilla-scented Peace candle that my niece Allison gave me last month. Out goes the worn blue mouse pad we've been using; in comes one with a brightly colored island scene, a souvenir from our last vacation.

Last but not least, I place a special angel beside the candle. She is one of a new line of angels I discovered in a gift store a few weeks before my diagnosis. Her name is Patience, and she sits hugging her knees to her chest with one arm, resting her chin on the other hand. I smile when I look at her. Perhaps she'll serve as a reminder for me to practice patience during the coming months of my new journey. Patience has never been my strongest virtue, but now I have an inner knowing that patience is one of the lessons I will learn, one of the blessings I will receive along the way.

Surveying the newly organized computer table with keen satisfaction, I gently touch the angel, then continue to roam the internet, looking for more connections to tighten the web of support I've already begun building for myself.

My brother Joe and his wife Karen drive up from Connecticut tonight to see *A Christmas Carol* with us at the theatre. I've decided to tell them about my cancer over dinner, but as we sit in the crowded steakhouse, sipping our margaritas and munching coconut shrimp, it is difficult to get to the place where I open my mouth and actually say the words. Joe has been talking about a recent visit to the doctor's office and when he finishes, I clear my throat, try to calm the butterflies in my stomach, and begin talking about my latest mammogram, the calcifications, the biopsy, the diagnosis. The words *I have breast cancer* still sound too drastic to me, so I use the words that Dr. Karp used.

They are quiet for a moment before asking a few questions. Dinner goes on as usual and our conversation changes to a myriad of other topics. Joe and Karen seem rather nonchalant about my news, and I'm wondering if maybe I've been a little too laid-back in the way that I told them. I'm actually feeling a little hurt that they didn't get all upset and make a big deal about it.

But after the show, as they're getting ready for the two-hour drive home, I'm struck with the intensity of the hugs they give me. They each hold me much, much longer and tighter than usual. They don't say anything, but I know now that they do indeed understand the seriousness of it all. There are tears in my eyes as I watch them drive away, but they are good tears. Tears of gratitude, of knowing that I am very much loved.

Sunday December 16

I email my brother John who lives three hours away in Connecticut. He is a social worker with his own counseling practice, and difficult to reach by phone. He replies quickly with both email and voicemail, reassuring me that he will add me to his Prayer Group's daily prayer list, and that he wants to be kept informed of my progress.

Later today I spend a long time talking with his wife Maryann, who asks just the right questions. She's an Oral Surgeon's Assistant, and her nearness to the medical profession makes me feel safe. She tells me that she had a cancerous melanoma on her leg several years ago. It was removed and she has to keep going back for checkups. She understands about hospitals and doctors. She understands the power of the word cancer.

I know I need to call my mother and tell her also, but I honestly don't know how. I just don't want to deal with her fears. I tell Jeff that I'll wait and tell her *after* the surgery but he won't hear of it. He's been so gentle with me, letting me make my own decisions about everything, so I'm surprised at the intensity of his insistence that she hear the news now. He offers to call her for me. I feel guilty but I let him do it. He tells me later that she asked a lot of questions and wrote everything down so she could tell her Prayer Group. There is no doubt in my mind that she is worried and upset, but I hope she'll find comfort in the fact that she and her friends can pray for me.

Monday December 17

This morning I talk with Dr. Karp and we set the date for the lumpectomy. January 3. I want to do it sooner (tomorrow wouldn't be soon enough) but he says he already has several surgeries scheduled for next week. When he hears the anxiety in my voice, he reminds me that these cancer cells have taken three or four years to become large enough to be seen with a microscope, and reassures me that they aren't going to grow very much in the next few weeks. That's easy for *him* to say, I think to myself as I hang up the phone. There aren't any cancer cells growing inside *his* body.

Tuesday December 18

Patience. A word that is increasingly taking on meaning for me as the days go by. I have a feeling that *Patience* is going to be my word for the year ahead. I found a collaged art print of the Asian symbol for patience and it is now framed and hanging in our bedroom, a constant reminder. I know intuitively that patience will be a key in the valuable lessons I'm already learning about the meaning of staying in the present moment. Having attempted this lesson before in my sporadic yoga and meditation practice over the years, I can see that breast cancer will be a more immediate and demanding teacher.

My mind is host to one colossal roller coaster ride of thoughts. There are whole stretches of time when my thinking goes like this: *The doctor isn't worried because we caught this so early. Look at how treatable it is. Look at how many people I've talked to and read about who've had cancer and survived it. Whew! I'm not going to die from this.* I am easily deceived into thinking I'm in for a smooth, easy ride. But every so often these thoughts collide with all the *what ifs* scurrying around in my brain. *What if the cancer has already spread to my lymph nodes? What if Dr. Karp has to take out all of the nodes under my arm and I have to be out of work for two weeks? What if I have to deal with lymphedema? What if he is wrong and the cancer has already spread to my bloodstream and they can't get it out? He was wrong when he told me that the calcifications were probably nothing; what if he's wrong this time too? What if the cancer cells come back? What if I'm one of the 45,000 women who die from this each year?* In the space of five seconds, my thoughts turn the ride into one that is bumpy, treacherous, scary, unsafe.

All of these *what ifs* feel like they're being juggled inside my head by a hyperactive clown at a not-so-funny circus. But there are way too many balls and they are moving too fast. I know I need to stay focused on positive thoughts, so when I notice the negative voices getting louder, I take a deep breath and slowly grab each ball, one at a time, and put it away. For now. I replace them with more life-affirming thoughts. *I am glad to be alive. Just for today I am healthy. All shall be well*. The maddening frenzy of the circus balls is replaced with simpler, more powerful thoughts.

This happens again tonight at the theatre when one of our Head Ushers tells me about his wife who is just finishing up her radiation treatments for breast cancer. He says how fatigued and "not herself" she's been the past two months. I can feel the fear building inside of me as I listen to him. My chest and throat are tight and my shoulders hunch up slightly in self-protection. The reality of my own diagnosis sweeps over me like a wave of bitter ocean water and for several long, awful moments, I feel like I might just drown in it.

But I don't. I consciously decide to shift my focus to something more positive. I acknowledge the fear and then move on to other thoughts- a good prognosis, a new opportunity for love and growth and healing. The fear subsides; the roller coaster ride evens itself out.

Wednesday December 19

This morning while browsing online, I order several books about breast cancer and breast health. I'm eager to read more about this new facet of my life, even though it has moved in and taken up residence without my consent. I instinctively know that the more information I have about this, the better I will feel. This has been true my whole life; whenever I'm faced with something new, my plan of attack is to read everything I can about it. I've always found comfort and safety and pleasure in books, and this will be no exception.

I also do a Google search using Dr. Karp's name and am pleased with what I find. He attained his medical degree in Canada. He spent several years in Virginia in a teaching/surgical position before moving here. It looks like he is one of the top breast surgeons in the business. When I look him up on the Lahey website, I discover that he is also the head of their new Breast Center. This fine assortment of facts fills me with gratitude. I feel more protected, more confident than before. There's something about seeing all of this information in black and white that lends additional weight to my anchor of safety.

Dr. Karp occupies my thoughts a lot today. I wonder why he left Virginia to come here. I wonder what he likes to do in his free time. My life is going to be in his hands on that operating table in a few weeks; I can't underestimate or be in denial about this simple yet complex fact. I should have the right to know something about him besides his medical credentials but I've never heard of anyone asking personal questions of their doctor. This is strange.

As I ponder this paradox, I decide it has something to do with boundaries. My experience with doctors has been completely limited to yearly physical exams and occasional flu-inspired visits. I've never had to think about boundaries in my relationships with doctors before. But this relationship with Dr. Karp is decidedly different because it comes attached to a cancer diagnosis. It comes with an assumption of being together for the "long haul" as he so eloquently stated last week. I'm wondering where the rules of this doctor-patient relationship are written. Has anyone ever thought of or written about this before? Am I the only patient who ever wanted to know her doctor in a more real and personal way?

Thursday December 20

Today I take a deep breath, sit down at the computer and send out a short email with my latest "news." I send it to just about everyone on my email list, asking for prayers and positive thoughts and support. It feels very strange to be writing an email like this, and yet it feels exactly right.

Friday December 21

I am completely overwhelmed with emotion as I read the return emails that are filling my Yahoo mailbox this morning.

My brother John forwards an email that he sent to his prayer group partners. In it he describes me as a *spiritual person who is drawing upon her faith at this time.* He reminds me that there are people all over the east coast who are praying for me, lifting me up through this whole experience.

JoAnn emails me a message of love and support. I'm so happy that she is my friend.

From our friends Eric and Valerie- *Our prayers are always with you but will be even more so over the next few months. If it's ok with you, we will tell Josh and Rachel so that you can be at the forefront of their prayers as well.* Gratitude sears my soul as I picture these dear children praying for me.

From my friend Hope in California- *I'm so sorry about your mammogram news. I know how scary this is as I went through much the same thing several years ago. I too had calcifications and they did a lumpectomy. I know it's no picnic but it sounds like your doctor is on top of things and you were fortunate to catch this in the early stages. Of course I'll pray for you and send good karma your way across the miles. This is more common than you know and you'll be surprised at how many women go through similar ordeals…… try to enjoy the holidays as much as you can. I'm thinking of you.* I've never met Hope but we share a love of collage, rubber stamp art, funny stories and David E. Kelly television shows. Now we have something else in common.

From my 20 year old nephew Peter in his college dorm room, two hours away- *Anything I can do to help you out, let me know. Love ya and miss ya lots.* It's been a long time since I've seen him and suddenly I miss him too. Peter also sends me a link to a website called *Hugs for the Cure*, which displays an animated teddy bear strolling across the screen. Suddenly the silly bear turns and looks right at me, walks towards me and opens his furry arms wide as if to give me a big hug. It is incredibly sweet and I'm embarrassed to admit how many times I click the replay button so I can see it again. Receiving this email feels like an extra helping of love.

From my former boss Sue, who has only recently come back into my life- *My thoughts and prayers are with you. I know you are a positive, bright woman who will take this time to heal using your divine intelligence. Let me know if there is anything I can do. I mean it! Are you taking any time off from work to focus on this? I will do some positive visualization exercises for you. Please keep me informed.* Ah, here is what Elizabeth was talking about, some genuine support from an unexpected source.

From my friend Connie in Illinois- *I am in shock to hear your news. I haven't been able to find the right words to say to you. You are probably taking this better than me.* I smile as I read this part of her email. She has gone deeply into the truth of her own response. Everyone who has read my email must be feeling the same shock, but she is the only one who has referred to it, and I appreciate her honesty.

From my 21 year old niece Stephanie in her college dorm room in New York City- *Thank you for letting us know. All my love is with you, and I'm very glad that the doctors feel this is treatable….. if there's anything you need, ever, even just a welcome ear, you know where to find me.* This message also brings tears to my eyes. My darling niece, kindred spirit, good with words and generous of heart, has said just the right things. A lot of people are telling me that everything's going to be okay, and that I'll be fine, but I can sense the worry underneath their cheerful words. Stephanie has said something different; she has reassured me that I am loved, and reaffirmed my positive outlook by reminding me that my cancer is treatable.

A few friends refer to the upcoming holidays and say they're glad I'll be surrounded by my family. I'm thankful for this too. I will exchange gifts with Jeff and his children on Christmas Eve, and on Christmas morning I'll drive the three hours to John (my brother) and Maryann's to spend the day with them. Mom, my brother Joe and his wife Karen will be there, along with Stephanie, Michael and Peter (my niece and nephews).

This morning is the final *Christmas Carol* production at the theatre. My friend George comes into the box office wearing his English Gentleman's costume prior to his first entrance. He waits until I hang up the phone, then opens his arms to me for a hug. He holds me for the longest time and without saying anything, I know he has read my email. It is very comforting, being held like this. He quietly asks me how I am. I feel touched, special. As he's leaving, he reminds me to be sure to let him know how I'm doing.

At one point I was thinking I wouldn't really like all the extra attention that having breast cancer was going to give me, but somewhere deep inside me I find that I'm actually enjoying it a little bit. For being the center of attention puts me in just the right place to receive this dazzling array of reminders of how very much I'm loved and treasured. And I can't help but think that this is going to be the fuel that eases me forward on my journey.

CHAPTER FIVE

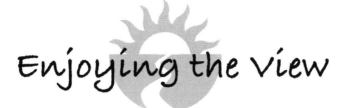

Enjoying the View

My barn having burned down, I can now see the moon.
— *Zen Koan*

Saturday December 22

It's amazing how quickly I seem to have gotten used to the fact that I have breast cancer. Was it only eleven days ago that I was crying hysterically over how much I didn't want this? Less than two weeks have passed and I have somehow been led to the edges of acceptance of it. Somehow I'm beginning to seek the blessings in it.

I wonder if this is just me and my positive mind-set, or is this true of any disastrous news? Can the human spirit simply adapt to anything? *Anything?*

I'm constantly aware of how I'm feeling about having breast cancer. It's like frequently feeling a child's forehead to be sure his temperature isn't spiking. What I'm noticing is that most of the time I actually feel okay about it. Not happiness exactly, but simply some hints and expectations of joy. I feel special, chosen, lifted. It's very strange, and it's the last thing I thought I would feel. I wonder if it's because so many people are now praying for me.

I've never been such a big focus for prayer because nothing much has ever been wrong with me before this.

Dr. Karp is also on my mind today, as are doctor-patient relationships in general. I wonder what other women have experienced in this area. Exactly how much can a woman ask her doctor about his own life? Where is the boundary? And what if I look at it from a doctor's perspective? Perhaps a doctor's boundary for closeness has to be tighter because of the fact that the patient may die. Maybe he can't get too close to his patients because that also means the danger of losing them.

And yet, isn't it natural for a woman to want to feel reasonably close to her breast surgeon? Her life is in his hands, literally. She's depending on his accumulated knowledge and wisdom. She's looking to him for a physical cure, for comfort and advice. Why can't she ask him what's going on in *his* life? Why can't she ask him if there's something *she* can do for *him*?

He's doing so much for me; isn't it natural to want to do something for him in return? I find myself wanting to bake him some cookies, or ask him if I can pray for him about something, or find the right words to make him laugh. I want to give him some kind of gift because of the gift he's giving me. Granted, I'm paying for this "gift" (I'm sure the bills will be rolling in very soon), but the gift of life that he's giving me goes beyond anything that money will buy.

Sunday December 23

Scooter, our hefty gray tiger cat, wakes me earlier than usual this morning. He lands with a thud on the bed and tentatively touches my cheek with his paw. He is gentle but insistent, and I reluctantly get up and go downstairs to let him out. Returning to sleep is impossible now, so I brew some decaf and carry it to my Quiet Room (a name given to my study by Jeff's brother Keith when we were building the house seven years ago). I put on some soft music and work on the five collage calendars that I started last week. One of them is for my mother, two are for friends, and the fourth is for me. The fifth calendar sits, still blank, on my desk. I haven't decided what to do with that one yet.

Coloring with the soft pencils is soothing to my spirit and occupies me for over an hour. When I've had enough, I carry the empty coffee mug downstairs and place it in the sink, savoring the quietness of the house with everyone still asleep. I consider going to church this morning. There's a 10:00 service in Topsfield. Perhaps I need to be there. I think of how church used to play such an important role in my life, and how now it's not part of my life at all. Part of me feels guilty and is telling me I *should* be going to church, *should* find a faith community, *should* have a priest I can turn to if I need one. But another part of me doesn't want to go to church this morning, needs something different. The other day, the thought crossed my mind that I may find what I need spiritually as a result of having breast cancer. A strange and unlikely thought, but intriguing nonetheless.

Instead of dressing and going to church, I settle down in the family room with another cup of decaf and our long-haired black cat Sasha on my lap. I pick up the first of the cancer books that I ordered online last week. *Spinning Straw Into Gold*, by Ronnie Kaye. The copyright date is ten years ago so I'm reading the medical information with a grain of salt, but the book is touching me deeply on many levels. The author talks about emotions, and body image, and the inner child.

She tells of a friend giving her a teddy bear in the hospital before her surgery. She asks the doctor if she can keep it with her in the operating room and he agrees. Oh, how I love this story! I have a few teddy bears sitting on the windowseat in our bedroom. One of them has been with me for forty years. At the ripe old age of five, I named him Timothy O'Shaughnessy MacGillicuddy Junior Esquire Pacheco. The sound of those words all strung together like that was music to my ears; I loved playing with words even then. The bear that sits beside him on our window seat is white and fluffy, larger, softer, more huggable. I've never given her a name but now I see that she needs one. Faith? Hope? Patience? Yes, that's it! Patience. I will give Timothy and Patience matching bright pink ribbons to wear around their necks. Perhaps I'll even take them with me to the hospital.

As I read the chapter on surgery, I begin thinking about my own body and am momentarily paralyzed by brief flashes of fear. The author had a mastectomy; I'm going to have a lumpectomy. One might think this would be less frightening, but it isn't. There is so much unknown, and this is the source of my biggest fear. What if the anesthesia makes me nauseous? Will I wake up sick to my stomach? What will Dr. Karp find when he takes out my sentinel node? If it is cancerous, will he then take out all of the nodes?

I feel the fear and acknowledge it, then turn it over to God, the

Universe, Spirit, Higher Power. It doesn't matter what name I give it; the effect is the same- a calming, deep release. An inner knowing that all really *shall* be well. This is the next part of my Journey and I'm learning to embrace it, fears and all.

Monday December 24

I find a quote today from Jennifer Louden that resonates throughout my entire being. It is about how acceptance leads to peace, which leads to gratitude, which is the basis for joy.

Her words sing to me because I have found that when I can be more truly accepting of my cancer (and all the dreaded ramifications that go with it), the peace that comes from not struggling with it makes me overflow with gratitude. And when I am feeling grateful, there is much more space for joy inside me.

It would be impossible to say that having cancer makes me happy. No, it's much deeper than that. More like touching an eternal wellspring deep inside of me, a mystical fountain of joy that's always right there below the surface, waiting for me to dive down into its rich warm healing waters.

I am slowly discovering that to experience this joy is a choice. First, I choose to accept the breast cancer. I accept that it is a part of me and that from now on my survival of it will forever be part of my self-definition. Accepting it doesn't mean that I am giving the cancer cells permission to wander throughout my body. It means simply accepting the fact that it has been slowly growing in my body for several years, that it is still here, now, in this moment. Accepting the cancer's presence is not the same as wanting it, nor does it mean I give it control.

Once I allow myself to accept the cancer (a choice I seem to need to make daily, sometimes hourly), then I find that I'm also facing my own mortality. I have to be comfortable with the fact that I'm going to die someday. I have to choose to accept this fact as well. We're all going to die. If I'm truly living with this fact, then every moment is more precious to me, more valuable, more keenly felt. And this leads to gratitude for each moment, each sensation, each sight, each feeling, each memory that is created. And that deep present-moment-living is the beginning of a deep, deep joy.

I'm reminded again of the prayer that I serendipitously found on the morning of my biopsy. *God, you are here. God, I am here.* This prayer is all about being in the moment. It's about remembering that I'm not alone. Spirit is with me, now, in this one moment. And then the next, and the next…

Perhaps now there are so many people praying for me that the power of this is lifting my spirit into realms I've never before been able to reach. This is the source of my feeling of being so totally supported, held, loved. This is the powerful energy fueling my explorations of joy at a time when I never would have expected joy to be possible.

Late this afternoon we exchange gifts with Jeff's children. There is laughter along with the rustle of wrapping paper and the spicy scent of warm cookies in the oven. For the first time in my life, I've kept Christmas simple. I ordered gifts online instead of wasting time and energy at the mall. We decorated just the tree instead of the entire house, and I baked two kinds of cookies instead of ten.

I sit back now and watch the kids laughing and talking in the glow of the soft tree lights, remembering Christmases when they were much younger, Christmases when we were so new at being a stepfamily. And instead of harshly judging myself a failure like I usually do when it comes to my thoughts about my role as a stepmother, I allow a new thought to form: we are a family, a good family, a stepfamily. We are the best family we know how to be. I've never had a thought like this before; my sense of stepfamily has almost always been clouded by my unrealistic expectations and self-doubt. I like this new thought and welcome it with an inner smile, feeling gratitude at the release it brings me.

Tuesday December 25

My Zen alarm clock chimes softly at 6:30 this morning. I kiss Jeff good-bye and begin the drive to Connecticut, singing along with the Christmas music on the radio. I stop in Rockville to pick up my mother. It's so difficult to drive the remaining hour with her pity lying on the front seat between us. Her solicitousness is not unexpected but it's upsetting nonetheless. This is the very reason why I didn't want to tell her about the diagnosis so soon: this pity that I knew I'd see in her eyes, in her every word and gesture. I want to scream *JUST TREAT ME LIKE NORMAL* but I don't because this is my mother and I don't think she knows how.

I remind myself gently that her good friend Marie died from breast cancer forty years ago. Because of this, the word "cancer" is probably capitalized and underlined in her mind, accompanied by red flags and flashing warning lights. I remind myself that I'm her child, and this has got to be a difficult thing for a mother to go through.

After a delicious dinner, my brothers fall asleep in the den and the rest of us play the word game *Taboo*. Laughter fills the room as the game goes on. I am grounded in the present moment with this, my beloved family. Their presence quietly seeps into my remembrance of who I am.

This whole afternoon reminds me of the Thornton Wilder play *Our Town*, which has touched my soul from the first time I read it in high school. When Emily says good-bye to life at the end of the play, she says these words- *Goodbye world, goodbye Grover's Corners, Mama and Papa. Goodbye to ticking clocks and my butternut tree and mama's sunflowers, food and coffee, new ironed dresses and hot baths and sleeping and waking up. Oh earth, you're too wonderful for anybody to realize you. Do any human beings ever realize life while they live it- every, every minute?*

I was only fourteen years old when I first read those words, and had made no acquaintance with death, but I instinctively knew that that soliloquy held the entire key to the meaning of life. As I heard Emily say those words in my young imagination, I grandly decided that *I* was going to live my life differently than she had. *I* was going to notice *every, every* detail. *I* was going to enjoy *every, every* minute of *my* life. When the end of *my* life came, I was not going to look back and realize I'd lived too quickly and not participated in it.

But then of course, life went on and I forgot the words and my life became a whirlwind of things to do, places to go. Yes, there were times when I paused, when I stood still and looked at the sky, but mostly Emily's words were forgotten. Every so often I would see *Our Town* on TV, or on stage, and the words would again ricochet out of an actress's mouth and into my soul, reminding me of the brevity of life, reminding me of the passion of my original intention.

Today, in this warm living room with my wildly funny, beautiful family, I'm reminded of Emily again and I smile to myself. The cancer is teaching me to open up and absorb how wonderful life really is. I've stopped and looked up at the sky more times this past week than I have in the last several years put together. Because of the cancer, I'm sitting here paying attention to these moments of laughter, appreciating Maryann's clever way with words, Peter's sense of humor, and Stephanie's creativity, instead of looking at my watch and wondering how much longer I should stay. Once again, I think with amusement that perhaps breast cancer will be the best teacher I've ever had, now that I am open to the lessons it brings.

When it's time for me to begin the long drive home, I find everyone lined up in the living room to hug me good-bye. Usually I have to run through the house and find each of them, but today is different and we all know it. I'm very close to tears in each of their familiar embraces, but when I get to Peter and he whispers in my ear that he's praying for me and wishing me luck next week, I give in and let the tears fall, and I am not ashamed. I am grateful with every ounce of my being to feel this much love from my family. I am fiercely grateful for each and every one of them.

Wednesday December 26

Today I put a note on the Survivor's Board with questions about the lumpectomy and sentinel node biopsy procedures. I mostly want to know what I should expect, explaining that I've never been in a hospital before as anything but a visitor.

I receive many responses on the board, and all of them reassure me that I'll be fine, that this kind of surgery entails minimal pain and an easy recovery. A woman named Dawn sends her reply to my email box instead of posting it on the board. She is 46, from Missouri, and was diagnosed just one day before me. She had two lumpectomies and the lymph node dissection before the surgeon got clean margins. She'll be starting chemo treatments in a few weeks and will have to have radiation after that. She's looking for an email buddy to go through treatments with and wonders if I'd be interested. I'm pretty sure I don't have to have chemotherapy, but I like the sound of having a buddy. All I asked for was some friendly advice and here is this woman who is offering me so much more. I email her back immediately and accept.

Thursday December 27

Today at work, my friend Joan tells me I'm handling all of "this" really well. I'm startled by her comment as we catch up on the filing, but I thank her and then murmur something about asking me how I'm handling it at 2 a.m. We laugh now but it's not really funny. The middle of the night is the hardest; the thoughts go buzzing through my mind like angry bees and there is no stopping them. They seem to gain power and mass in that deep darkness lit only by the neon numbers on the alarm clock.

I break down in tears tonight after supper for no particular reason other than I'm feeling a little sorry for myself. Jeff comes to my side and holds me, strokes my hair and tells me for the thousandth time that we're going to get through this together. I apologize later for crying on his shoulder yet again and his response is balm to my tired, sore spirit. *Who else's shoulder are you going to cry on?* Of course, this starts the tears rolling again but now my tears are laced with gratitude.

What on earth would I do without this man? I already know from the women online that there are men who leave when breast cancer moves in with them. There are boyfriends, girlfriends, lovers, partners, and husbands who run away, who shun the disfigured body, who cannot deal with the changes, the doctors, the treatments, the tears. I hold Jeff a little more tightly. There are men who leave, but I've been blessed with one of the men who stay. And not just a man who stays, but one who embraces, comforts, and continues to love.

Friday December 28

Last week I ordered a raku pendant online, and today it arrives in the mail. It's pretty, a soft weathered sage green with coppery highlights, and engraved with the Chinese symbol for patience. I loop the black silk cord over my head and reverently touch the clay. I'll be wearing this every day as a reminder of the lessons I'm learning on this new journey.

Tonight we drive to Cambridge for dinner at *Fire and Ice* with Harvey and Elaine. Jeff knows Harvey from a former job, and we've been out to dinner with them a few times. Most of the evening I'm able to forget about the cancer. There is laughter and good conversation, excellent food and cold beer. Then Harvey starts asking me questions about my doctor, about the surgery. I should probably be annoyed that he's interrupting my "normal" evening out with reminders of the disease, but his questions are genuine and to the point. He isn't showering me with platitudes about how everything is going to be all right. Both he and Elaine are sincerely interested, but not full of pity. I find this comforting, like finding a shady tree to rest under after climbing a steep hill. It's like they haven't forgotten who I am in the midst of the crisis.

After dinner, they each hug me closely. I'm startled but touched by this show of affection. Harvey tells me they'll be thinking of me next week, and tells Jeff to call him as soon as the surgery is over. The gesture and the words warm me inside and out. There is indeed support and love coming from the most unexpected places. And to think my first inclination was not to tell anyone that I have breast cancer!

Tuesday January 1

Jeff falls asleep early on New Year's Eve, but I choose to stay awake. At the stroke of midnight I'm sitting in my favorite rocking chair, welcoming the New Year in. Alone except for a warm, sleeping Sasha on my lap. Her sweet presence permeates my body and soul. The first hour of 2002 finds me praying, meditating, and taking a warm bubble bath by soft pink candlelight. I pray that the year ahead has more of these clarifying, indulgent moments in store for me. Let this new year be full of Patience, Joy, Love, and Letting Go. Not only in spite of the breast cancer, but because of it.

Wednesday January 2

This morning Dr. Karp spends fifteen minutes with me on the phone, answering my questions about the surgery tomorrow. The conversation fills me with confidence. I believe that I have the best doctor and that I will be at the best hospital. This certainty dispels a great deal of my fear and worry.

As I lie in bed tonight, seeking sleep, I decide to do a visualization exercise. This was once an integral part of my spiritual life, but I've not meditated this way in several years.

I close my eyes, focus on my breathing, and imagine the most peaceful space I know. It is the spacious living room of a house by the ocean, close enough to hear the waves crashing on the shore through the open windows. I picture myself lying on a long hospital stretcher in the middle of this room. All is quiet. Moonlight softens the darkness of this sacred space. I feel safe here, peaceful, at home.

As my eyes acclimate to the dark, I look around me and realize that everyone I know (and have ever known) is here. Everyone. They form a wide circle around me. I get up from the stretcher and walk around the circle slowly, facing each person, touching each one in some way, letting them touch me. The feeling of intimacy and love is breathtaking, and I allow it to wash over and through me as completely as the ocean waves embrace the sand outside the windows.

Jeff is here, with his three children- Amanda, Jeffrey and Merri. My father is here and it doesn't surprise me to see him even though he passed away eight years ago. There are others: My mother. Jeff's mother Connie. My friends from the theatre. Jeff's brothers and sister and their families. My brothers and their wives. My precious nieces and nephews. Allison hands me a single wild iris, my favorite flower. Randy, Doug, Greg, and Chris are here, the Episcopal priests on my journey who have ministered to me the most over the years. Elizabeth and Dawn are standing together away from the others. I've never met them but I recognize them instantly. JoAnn and her husband Jim have come to join us as well as Lori and her daughter Rebekah. Val and Eric are here with Josh and Rachel; my heart warms at their sweet hugs. Rachel smoothes my hair back from my face, like a mother would comfort a child and I am indeed comforted. George and Jay, my actor friends, are over there on the far side of the circle, serenading me quietly with the song Agony *from* Into the Woods. *I laugh out loud when I recognize what they are singing.*

I turn to go back to the stretcher and see my three beloved cats. Sasha is curled up at the bottom, where my feet will be when I lie down. Scooter is stretched out with his tiger tummy facing up on the right side of the stretcher, just the right place for me to cuddle him. And Minnie is sitting smack in the middle of the stretcher, meowing loudly as is her custom, almost (but not quite) in tune with George and Jay. I pick up her soft little gray and white body and hand her over to Rachel for safekeeping while I lie back down, surrounded by family, friends and cats.

Closing my eyes, I consciously absorb all of this love and carry it back with me to the reality of my bedroom where my husband lies snoring softly beside me. I decide that this is the image I'm going to take with me tomorrow when I lie in the operating room awaiting my surgery. I will visualize this healing circle of people who know and love me. And I know without a doubt that whatever happens, all will be well.

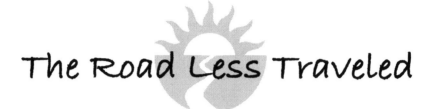

CHAPTER SIX

The Road Less Traveled

Teach us…
That we may feel the importance of every day,
of every hour, as it passes.

— from a prayer by Jane Austen, circa 1811

Thursday January 3

This is it. Surgery today. The alarm is set but I wake up long before it chimes its Zen tones. A sense of anticipation and dread swirl through me as I shower and dress.

There are butterflies in my stomach when Jeff and I walk into Lahey Clinic this morning. It's not quite 7:30; the lobby is empty, the player piano silent. I smell fresh coffee and tuna from the small cafeteria on the main floor. When I get to the lab for my blood work, there are several people already there, waiting on the straight gray chairs. My name is the first one called and the blood tests are quick and painless.

The lobby area of the Outpatient Surgery wing is crowded. Jeff finds us two empty seats and settles himself in with his briefcase open on his lap.

I'm nervous as I sit beside him, but I breathe deeply and slowly, attempting to calm myself. I pick up a woman's magazine from the low table in the corner and flip through it, looking at (but not really seeing) the glossy pictures.

Finally a cheerful nurse calls my name and I follow her behind the curtain. This isn't what I expected at all. We're walking down a very wide corridor. There is much activity, seemingly in defiance of my every effort to be calm. Nurses walk quickly, almost running; patients are ambling past us; men and women in blue scrubs and plastic hats stand in small groups here and there, talking animatedly and in normal tones. Why do I think they should be whispering? Perhaps I've watched too many episodes of *Chicago Hope*.

The nurse leads me to one of the little rooms that is separated from the corridor by a pale green curtain. She is calling it an "ambulatory suite" and I'm amused at the euphemism. It certainly sounds lovely but this isn't my idea of a suite. There is a bed on wheels in the middle of the room, an IV stand, a plain white table, and a tall cupboard. White metal blinds cover the tall windows which overlook the highway below.

She snaps a pale green plastic identification bracelet on my wrist, then instructs me to take off all of my clothing, and gives me a large plastic bag to put everything in. The bag has my name on it in large black letters. She swishes the curtain shut behind her and I do as I was told, then put on the pale blue hospital gown and lie down on the bed, consciously breathing slowly and deeply.

In a few minutes, a different nurse comes in, enveloped in a bustling aura of kindness. She hangs a plump clear plastic bag from the IV pole, plays around with the veins on my right hand, then connects me to the IV with a few swift movements and tubes. She explains that this is to keep me hydrated. They call Jeff from the waiting area and he joins me as we wait for the volunteer who is going to wheel me around to my various appointments in other parts of the hospital.

I certainly wasn't expecting to be hooked up to an IV so soon. Dr. Karp never mentioned this. I wonder how I look to my husband as I lie here, naked under this thin ugly gown, not wearing makeup, in a starkly lit hospital "suite" with an IV bottle dripping clear liquid into my veins. I'm glad there isn't a mirror nearby. If I could see myself now, I might truly be frightened. I might be forced to admit exactly why I'm here.

A volunteer named Veronica arrives, smiling and jovial. She's an older, heavyset woman with gray and black curls framing her wide face. She wheels me deftly through the halls and elevators, Jeff following closely behind. I joke with her about where she got her driver's license. She takes me first to Nuclear Medicine where I am x-rayed and then injected with radioactive dye, then x-rayed again.

After this, Veronica wheels me over to Mammography. She pats my arm and says that someone will come and get me when they are ready for me, and that she'll be back when I am done. Jeff kisses me good-bye before leaving to do some errands. And here I am, suddenly alone.

I had thought I'd be able to maintain an illusion of control, but I see now how ridiculous this is. There is no more illusion. I have absolutely *no* control. I'm lying pretty much naked on a gurney in a hospital hallway with an IV attached to my right hand. I can't get up and take a walk. I can't even go to the bathroom without help. It's impossible to turn around and see what's going on behind me. I feel like a prisoner. I feel very alone. I'm close to tears now, as this powerlessness invades my idea of who I am. But I'm not going to give in to the fears and the loneliness. I concentrate once more on my breathing. I picture the circle of family and friends surrounding me, feel their warmth and love. This powerful image takes the edge off of my isolation, takes the panic away from my fear.

After twenty minutes, a short pleasant-faced woman comes over to me. Her name badge identifies her as Mary, Mammography Technician. She helps me off the gurney so I can walk into the room where the wire insertion is going to take place. My memories of this room are already filled with stress and fear because it's the same space where the radiologist told me that I needed to see a breast surgeon.

Mary sits beside me and chats about the weather, what she did for New Year's, my job, her favorite shows at the theatre. This bright chatter goes on for several minutes before the radiologist comes in. I smile uneasily at him, and wonder if he remembers telling me about the calcifications.

Mary eases the gown off my shoulders, apologizing because it's chilly in here. I stay seated for the mammogram, which feels very odd as I've always stood for mammograms in the past. My poor left breast (already tender from PMS) is squished many times for several different views. She apologizes every time she takes another picture. I am trying once again to focus on my breath, but it's impossible to ignore the pain.

Mary is now standing behind me, her warm solid hands on my shoulders. The comfort this touch gives me makes me want to weep. We continue to talk, about her dog, my cats, and our favorite movies. This is taking much longer than I ever thought possible. At one point I ask her if she's going to help the doctor with the procedure, and she tells me she's just here to keep me company. I look at her in bewilderment. She isn't joking. Surely she must be some kind of angel. I cannot imagine going through this without her, distracting me with her perky chatter, massaging my shoulders, reminding me that I have a life separate from this new one that's been thrust upon me.

The wire insertion is painful. Some of the bright turquoise dye spills onto my hand. I smile when I see it and tell them this is one of my favorite colors. Mary says it's a good thing I like it because I'm going to be peeing in this color for the next 24 hours. We laugh together at this, and some of the pain dissolves.

Veronica comes back when this procedure is over and wheels me through the hospital's maze of corridors, into a different room in the Ambulatory Surgery wing. I amuse myself by watching the nurses and doctors walking past my room. They're dressed alike in smoky blue loose pants and tops. A few of them are wearing pale blue plastic bonnets but most of them are wearing more stylish scrub caps. One of them is dark blue with silver and gold stars. I really like that one. One is embroidered with brightly colored dogs and cats. That's my second favorite.

I entertain myself with this fashion parade for several minutes until a handsome young man studying a clipboard enters my suite and introduces himself as my anesthesiologist. As he shakes my hand, I'm thinking he looks the same age as my nephews who are still in college. He asks me how I'm feeling, then waits patiently for my answer. I tell him I'm ready for a nap and he laughs out loud. I like that he does this. He pulls out my chart and tells me he's ready for a nap too. I tell him it's not acceptable for my anesthesiologist to be napping on the job. He laughs again and I'm grateful for the sound of it.

He's wearing one of the plain blue plastic scrub caps, so I ask him why he doesn't have a more colorful one like everyone else here. He tells me he's not a slave to fashion and this time it's my turn to laugh. Then the questions begin. My medical history. Allergies. Pain. He makes several notes on my chart while I reel off my answers like I'm on a television quiz show.

After he leaves, Dr. Karp wanders into my room. He comes right up to me, lays his hand on my shin and asks how I'm doing. I find his touch comforting somehow, although it is light and brief.

I admire his bright green surgical cap which has a tropical jungle scene imprinted on it in bold beautiful colors. He grins and thanks me, touching his hand to the cap. He tells me he has another cap at Lahey Burlington that is similar to this one but it has fish all over it. He really wanted one with *carp* on it but had to settle for trout and salmon. Still, he likes the one with the fish on it better than the one he's wearing now. He shrugs and grins, tells me he'll be back, disappears around the corner.

Dr. Karp seems a little more human to me now and that makes me happy. I can hear the wheels in my brain spinning already. There *is* something that my doctor needs, something special that he wants. I decide right here and now to find him a surgical cap with carp on it. Not that I have any idea what carp look like, because I don't. But I do know my way around the internet and I know that I can find pretty much anything I want if I set my mind to it. And I will set my mind to this.

It's almost noon when several medical personnel finally bustle into my room. One of them kicks free the brake on my bed and they wheel me down the hall, through a pair of large steel swinging doors. There are several operating rooms down this hallway and I'm wheeled into one of them. It's not as big as I thought it would be. I wince at all the bright lights and shiny metal. The staff wheels me up beside the black table in the center of the room and I clumsily manage to shift myself onto it.

There's a large white board on the wall opposite me; it makes me smile to see my name written on it in big red letters. I'm sure it's there for the medical staff but I like being reminded of who I am. There is something sacred to me about this, my name in huge letters right in front of me.

Dr. Karp comes up to me, touches my ankle lightly. Again, I'm comforted by this touch which seems to ground me in both body and spirit. In my experience, the doctor rarely touches the patient, except to examine the area of the body that presents the illness. This touch seems simply meant for comfort, a reminder that he is present.

One of the nurses asks me if I have any allergies and I begin to recite them, but Dr. Karp is already writing them on the board under my name. He has remembered every one of them from the first time I told him, and this comforts me even more than his touch.

I really don't want to see any more, so I close my eyes and begin imagining my circle of family and friends. I picture each one of them right there in the O.R. with me. Sasha and Scooter are warming my body on the table, and I can see Minnie in Rachel's arms nearby. I imagine their faces but it's their love that is calming me. I know that right now they're praying for me, beaming good thoughts my way. I'm surrounded from within and without by this feeling of genuine nurturing.

Dr. Karp's voice interrupts my meditation. He is asking the nurses where the probe is. Probe? What probe? This sparks my curiosity but I keep my eyes closed. Maybe I don't really want to know. After a few minutes I realize that the room is filled with strange music. It sounds otherworldly, like it's coming from another planet, vaguely reminiscent of the tones from the alien mothership in *Close Encounters of the Third Kind*. I keep my eyes closed, still fearful of what I might see if I open them, and ask Dr. Karp if he plays this kind of space music in the O.R. all the time. Suddenly everyone in the room is laughing and I open my eyes to see what is so funny.

He's sitting beside me on a stool with wheels, and next to him is a square machine that looks like a Geiger counter. This is the machine that shows him exactly where the radioactive dye is in my body, and he shows me how it works. He moves the probe (a long metal forklike instrument) close to my breast and its metallic beeps scurry all over the scale. He moves it away from me and it simply hums quietly.

Now the anesthesiologist tells me to close my eyes and breathe deeply. I do as I'm told, totally content that I've managed to make everyone laugh right before my surgery.

I'm awake again, just barely, in what seems like five seconds. I hear the movements and sounds of several people around me. One of the women is saying in an agitated voice that she had to put in another IV. Another female voice is telling me the surgery is over. As I fade in and out of consciousness, I listen for Dr. Karp's voice but all I hear are women. My lips are dry and there's a strange metallic taste in my mouth. My eyelids feel like they're glued shut; it's impossible to open them.

I'm licking my lips and clearing my throat a lot, also wiggling my toes. This seems to be the only movement possible to me right now.

After a while I realize there's only one other person in the room with me. It takes a great deal of effort but I manage to open my eyes.

I'm in a small room with a wide opening that is across from the nurse's station. The room itself is dark but I can see bright sunlight peeking through the vertical blinds. The nurse is about my age and she smiles to see me awake. She tells me I've been here for almost an hour and a half. I can see the clock across the hall. It says 2:45. So it's been three hours since they wheeled me into the OR. Absolutely amazing. My sense of time is completely distorted.

The nurse starts talking to me about sitting in the big blue chair that's over by the window, but I'm seriously doubtful. Right now all I want to do is close my eyes and submit to the call of slumber.

She cranks my bed up several inches and the desire for slumber goes just a little further away. I ask for Jeff and soon he's by my side, grinning and holding my hand. I feel full of gladness to see him. His presence brings me some necessary groundedness. This is real. This is home. I am awake. The surgery is over and my husband is beside me. All is well.

Jeff tells me that Dr. Karp told him he's pretty sure he got all of the cancerous cells with clean margins, and that the sentinel node looked clear when they tested it in the OR but he is sending it to the lab to be certain. I breathe a sigh of relief and continue holding Jeff's hand.

Two hours tick slowly by before I manage to walk the short distance to the chair by the window. The nurse has opened the blinds and I'm looking out onto Route 128. Car headlights are starting to burn brightly against the silvery dusk. With Jeff's help I put on my bra (I bought one just for this; it's a size bigger, all cotton, and hooks in the front) and finish getting dressed. The nurse gives me a sheet of post-op instructions and a prescription for Tylenol with codeine in case I feel any pain.

Jeff wheels me down to the lobby where the player piano music is lilting and cheerful. I drink in the music, and the normal sight of people coming and going, all the while feeling still and centered both inside and out.

I can hardly believe the day is over. I'm extremely talkative on the ride home; Jeff listens quietly to my chatter. I tell him the story about the surgical caps and the anesthesiologist who refuses to wear a colorful one. It feels so good to be sitting upright in a moving car. I feel normal. But I also notice a vague loneliness washing over me like a cool damp rain. There's no way that Jeff can really know what I've just been through. No way he can really understand. I feel a sudden desire to talk about it with someone who knows.

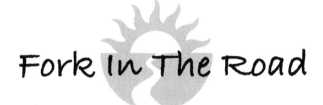

CHAPTER SEVEN

Fork In The Road

One never goes so far as when one doesn't know where one is going.
— Johann Wolfgang von Goethe

Friday January 4

I have slept more deeply than usual. Lying flat on my back, unable to shift to either side, my mind and body are still lethargic from the anesthesia. I'm pleased that I haven't had to take the codeine. My breast feels incredibly sore. The extra-strength Tylenol seems to be keeping the pain at bay.

Jeff kisses me good-bye, tells me he made me a few tuna sandwiches and put them in the fridge for me. I am touched, blessed, by this small act of kindness. It's been 12 hours since I laid down, so I get up after he leaves. It feels so good to stretch my legs. I'm not supposed to take a shower yet, so I splash some cold water on my face and change the gauze pad that's tucked up against the wound on my breast.

The house is utterly still. Sasha has spent the long night curled at my feet, her customary position. She is now sitting, queenlike, at the foot of the bed, carefully washing her face with her right paw, but keeping an eye on me at the same time. I sit beside her, stroke her velvety fur, allow her sandpaper tongue to caress my hand. Then I slowly walk down the stairs. My legs still feel a little wobbly and my head is a little fuzzy, but I feel gloriously happy that I'm home where I belong and the surgery is over.

I open the front door which lets in not only the biting cold January air but Scooter, who meows at me indignantly and then swaggers to the dining room doorway where he awaits his food dish alongside Sasha. Minnie joins them from her corner bed in the living room. I relish the familiar movements of opening the can of cat food, listening to their enthusiastic purrs as they brush up against me, purring with gusto as they lick the bowls clean.

Watching them eat, I realize I'm ravenous. I take an English muffin and a glass of apple juice upstairs with me and sit down at the computer. My first priority is sending emails to Dawn and Elizabeth. I tap out yesterday's story while munching my breakfast. It feels good to be telling my story to women who've been through exactly what I'm going through now. I don't feel as lonely as I did last night.

I also sum up my surgery experience in four paragraphs and send it out as a group email to family, friends, people at work. It feels good to be connecting with them also. Thank goodness for email. I'm definitely too tired for lots of phone calls or visits, but the internet is allowing me to stay in touch with the people who are important to me without compromising my recovery time.

Later in the afternoon, the doorbell interrupts my nap. Soon I hear my stepson Jeffrey thumping up the stairs. He appears at the door with a beautiful flower arrangement. It's a sage green wicker basket filled with a soft explosion of evergreens interspersed with brightly colored spring flowers. He hands me the card and places the arrangement on my nightstand. The flowers are from John and Maryann, and I smile while reading the note.

I breathe in the fresh pine scent as Jeffrey picks up several things that have fallen off the bed. He asks if I need anything else. My heart softens. For the last few years, Jeffrey and I have stayed out of each other's way, for the safety and sanity of the household. His life choices and daily habits have seemed unacceptable to me, and yet my voice in these matters has been unwelcome. I am relieved now, for in this brief moment, I see a glimpse of the Jeffrey I knew ten years ago: a kind, sweet, thoughtful boy, now on his way to manhood. I smile as I thank him, and am truly grateful for his presence.

Saturday January 5

I sleep deeply once again and don't awaken until 11:00. Jeff is gone, the room is dark, and I feel lonely and depressed for no particular reason. I sit up in bed and suddenly find myself crying. It feels good to let the tears out instead of holding them back, but I'm shocked by the intensity of the feelings. Maybe this is a result of the anesthesia? I think I read something about this somewhere. When the tears stop, I walk slowly and stiffly to the bathroom, wash my face, brush my teeth. It's amazing, the power of clean teeth to brighten one's outlook on life. I can take a shower today but don't feel like expending any more energy right now. To tell the truth, I'm feeling a little sorry for myself. I turn on the TV, climb back under the covers, and flip through the channels to see what's on.

My brother Joe calls and wants to know if I'm up for a visit from him and Stephanie tomorrow. I really don't feel like seeing anyone, but I know that I'll probably feel better if I spend some time with family, so I tell him yes.

I get back into bed, looking forward to indulging in some more self-pity, hiding out under the covers, but Jeff comes in with the mail. There are several cards for me and I find myself smiling at them in spite of myself. There also is a huge box from Hope. I open it with growing curiosity, to find the biggest, softest teddy bear I've ever seen. It's love at first sight. He's at least two feet tall and is the most beautiful shade of amber honey. There is a red and white checked bow tie around his neck. I toss the box on the floor and hug him to me, more tears leaking onto his agreeable head. He's just the right size for hugging and I don't let go of him for several hours.

Later, Jeff and I watch a few of the *Vicar of Dibley* videos that I bought right after Christmas just for this purpose. They work their hilarious magic; I find myself laughing out loud in spite of myself.

Late in the afternoon the doorbell rings and this time Jeffrey carries up a beautiful dish garden from my friends at the theatre. It seems that no matter how hard I try, I'm not able to stay depressed for very long today.

Sunday January 6

I make myself get up around 9:00 even though I'd much rather stay in bed. I'm still sluggish from the anesthesia, but aware of the need to make myself presentable before Joe and Stephanie arrive. I take a much-welcomed shower and wash my hair for the first time in four days. This in itself makes me feel better. I dry off carefully, change the gauze dressing again and put on some makeup after I get dressed. I look at myself in the mirror. Yes, that's me. So much the same, yet so much is different now.

When Joe and Stephanie walk in the door after their two hour drive, I'm immediately glad to see them. Their hugs and presence are just what it takes to remind me that I'm loved and cherished by others besides my husband and cyberspace friends. That my brother and niece have made this effort to reach out to me beyond email, beyond a phone call, touches me deeply, grounds me into a different sort of reality: a reality of long deep love, a reality that only my family of origin can give me.

Stephanie gives me a handmade box that she decoupaged with beautiful green art papers. On top of the box is the Chinese symbol for health. I decide to put this by the computer, beside the peace candle and soft glass lamp. A fitting object for my newly created sacred space. A constant reminder of my own responsibility for my health. A constant reminder of Stephanie's love.

After they leave, I zip up my winter coat, and head for the library and grocery store. It feels good to be out in the fresh winter air, but when I'm home again, I'm all too happy to put on my nightgown and climb back under the blankets for a nap.

Tuesday January 8

I go back to work today and am immediately welcomed with huge hugs from Joan and John. Lisa comes up from Systems and sits beside me for a few minutes. She genuinely wants to know how I'm feeling and what's next for me. She tells me her dad had throat cancer eleven years ago, went through the chemo and the radiation, and is fine today. I didn't know this, and the knowing makes me glad. Her story brings me hope as it reminds me once again that more people survive cancer than not.

It's good to be back at the theatre, but I feel changed somehow, even though everything here is exactly the same. I've grown so much in the last month, more than I ever thought or imagined possible. My priorities are different now, my whole life perspective is different. Right now we're working on reseating our subscribers for the upcoming Broadway musical season. I usually love this part of my job but right now it feels rather empty.

I feel as though my life is never ever going to be the same again. It may look on the outside like everything is the same (except for these two small scars), but on the inside I know that I'm forever and indelibly changed. Breast cancer has entered and invaded my life; it has transformed me and not just on a cellular level. There is fear, but there is also blessing. There is pain, but there is also joy. I'm learning to let go of things much more quickly than I ever thought possible.

Tonight after supper I ask Jeff about his feelings during my surgery. I've been curious about this. Was he scared, upset, worried upon seeing me in the hospital with the IV tubes in me? Has he actually realized that I had something inside my body that could take my life before I'm ready to give it up? He seems thoughtful about my questions, and pauses before answering. He tells me that he didn't like seeing me on that hospital gurney, but he believes I'm going to be okay because of the positive facts, statistics and expectations that Dr. Karp has given us.

He holds me, although it is uncomfortable because my breast is still sore, as is the incision from the sentinel node biopsy. I relax against his body, allowing his affirmation to fill me, to remind me that *all shall be well, and all shall be well, and all manner of thing shall be well.* At least for this moment, which is all I really have. *All is well.*

Wednesday January 9

I am carefully studying a subscriber's request for different theatre seats for the season. Outside, in spite of the chilling wind, the early afternoon sun rakes its way across the parking lot and I have to close the blinds halfway to deflect the brightness. I sip some water, flip through a few computer screens, looking for just the right seats that will make these longtime customers happy. The effort, the challenge totally absorbs me. Beside me, John is working on similar requests from subscribers; across the room, Joan and Dina and Jocelyn are doing the same.

My phone rings and I answer absent-mindedly, still frowning at the screen. "North Shore Music Theatre, this is Anne."

"Anne, it's Dr. Karp!" The energy in his voice pulls my eyes away from the computer screen and I find myself staring at the phone instead. It's been almost a week since the surgery….is the pathology report finally ready? I have actually forgotten all about it, figuring no news is good news.

He asks me how I am and if it's okay to call me at work. We're talking about breast cancer here, aren't we? What difference does it make if I'm at work? I realize I'm holding my breath now and as he begins to speak, I realize why.

It seems that no news isn't necessarily good news. The pathology report from the surgery shows precancer cells on the perimeter of the 2.2 centimeter lump that he removed, which means I'm going to have to have surgery again, so he can open up the incision and take out more tissue, trying once again for clean margins. I grab a ticket envelope from the small stack beside my computer and begin scribbling notes as he talks. There's no way I can remember all of this without writing it down.

And then there's more. He didn't just take out one sentinel node, he took out two, and the second node has a microscopic cancer cell on it. This means that, not only am I going to have to have the full lymph node dissection, I'm going to have to have the chemo as well as the radiation.

This is absolutely the last thing I expected. Absolutely the last. He says he's sorry and asks if I have any questions for him now. I can think of only one: when will this next surgery be? He thinks probably the last week in January or the first week in February. I wonder aloud if it can really wait that long and he reminds me that these cancer cells grow very slowly, then assures me that a few weeks is not that long to wait. Easy for him to say, I'm thinking. He tells me he'll call me as soon as the surgery date is scheduled.

I hang up the phone and stare out the window, aware once again of movement and sound around me. Everyone is still working. No one seems to notice that I've just gotten off the phone with my doctor. Either that, or they are simply allowing me some space and privacy. If this is true, I'm grateful because I realize I'm about to cry. I get up slowly from my chair and head for the ladies room.

Once there I do cry for a little while, in the handicapped stall which allows more space than the others. I plop myself down on the floor and let myself cry quietly for a few minutes. I'm feeling more than a little angry and hurt, betrayed by my own body, abandoned by my own "positive attitude."

More cancer. My brilliant breast surgeon didn't get all of the cancer, and there is still some of it in my body, my breast, my lymph nodes. Precancer. Microscopic. Does it really matter how tiny it is? Am I supposed to comfort myself with the fact that what remains is miniscule? Somehow I cannot. I've been fooling myself with the assumption that The Cancer was completely eradicated and that the worst of my problems were over, but this conversation with my doctor has been a slap in the face slamming me back into reality. I still have breast cancer. It still invades my body and somehow, *somehow,* I have to summon the energy and strength and courage to continue this journey even though it's going to take me places where I don't want to go.

Eventually I blow my nose on some toilet paper and hoist myself up to look in the mirror. My face is flushed and my eyes are a little red, but I look okay. I have to go back into that office; I have to finish out the afternoon no matter how much I'd rather stay here on this hard black bathroom floor and cry. There are subscribers awaiting new seats, there are donations to be processed, there are jokes to be shared with Joan and John and Dina and Jocelyn. Sitting here in the bathroom will accomplish nothing. I must go back.

As I take my seat again, John leans over, his eyes kind and searching. "Are you okay?" he asks gently. I nod, biting my lower lip to keep back the tears, and tell him I'll be all right. I can't quite bring myself to tell anyone this new twist in the story. If there's one thing I've learned about myself in the past few months, it's that I have to give myself a little time to absorb news like this before I can speak it aloud to someone else. So I allow myself this time and space, continuing to sit at my desk, changing subscribers' seats, one renewal form after another, until the setting sun changes the sky to a deep golden orange behind the trees on the far side of the parking lot.

CHAPTER EIGHT

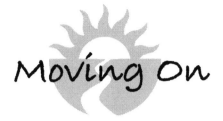

Moving On

*How can a man's life keep its course
if he will not let it flow?*

— *Tao Te Ching*

Monday January 14

I leave work before noon today, heading for Lahey for meetings with all of my doctors. Jeff meets me in the noisy hospital cafeteria and we have lunch together before going up to the third floor.

There are four breast cancer patients here today, and it startles me when I recall that *I* am one of them. Will I ever get used to this new label?

The nurse in my examining room spends fifteen minutes taking my medical history, then instructs me to undress from the waist up (why am I not surprised?). I reluctantly take the gown from her hands, disappointed that I won't be able to wear my favorite sweater because I feel so much more like *myself* when I'm wearing it. This gown, this perennial object of hospital fashion, takes away some of my identity, my uniqueness, and instantly labels me "patient." I don't like this feeling at all. It puts me at a distinct disadvantage in this day full of doctors. They of course will probably be wearing white jackets but at least their shirts and ties and blouses will be showing underneath, some semblance of personality will still be allowed to show through. This piece of gray cotton totally negates my personality, makes me feel like I'll be meeting these doctors in a subordinate position somehow. But I don't protest. I sigh deeply and dutifully shrug into it after the nurse leaves. I decide I'll have to focus a little harder on remembering who I am, on finding ways to be *myself* with these doctors. I passionately wish for them to *see* me as I am, a woman with a life, a family, hobbies and interests beyond breast cancer.

I leave my favorite turquoise sweater folded carefully on the table beside me so I can see it. The color alone cheers me. I lift my favorite beaded necklace over my head and wrap it several times around my left wrist. This was handmade at Kripalu, a yoga retreat center in the Berkshires, and I bought it there fifteen years ago. It's made of hundreds of small forest green and rose colored semiprecious stones with tiny gold spacer beads between each one. I've always felt protected when I've worn it although I have no idea why. I understand that wearing it around my neck while all of these doctors are examining my breasts is not a good idea, so I've created another way to keep it visible and close to my body.

Now Jeff and I are waiting. I'm much more talkative than usual because I'm feeling keyed-up and hopeful. Keyed-up because I know that today I'll be meeting my medical oncologist and my radiation oncologist plus the social worker who runs breast cancer survivors' support group, and I'm eager to meet all of them. Hopeful because I know that I'm in a place of healing, a place where "problems" like mine seem easily solved. I like being this near to the healing, to the healers. It makes me feel safe.

When I went to the bathroom earlier, I walked by the conference room where my three doctors and the social worker are now sitting, going over my (and the other women's) medical records. All of my information is in that room with them- pathology reports, x-rays, mammograms, blood work results, anecdotal records...etc. After reviewing our histories and reports, each doctor will visit each of us for as long as we want. Then they'll go back to the conference room and make notes about us, talk to the other doctors, share notes and ideas about treatment plans while they're all in the same place. I like this whole concept immensely. It feels like family somehow, to be doing it this way. Even more, I like the idea of meeting my other doctors this far ahead in the process. And I know from my postings on the breast cancer survivor's bulletin board that some women don't meet their treatment doctors until the day their treatment begins, so I'm glad that Lahey's process is different.

The first to knock on the door is Dr. Morganstern, my medical oncologist. He will be responsible for my chemotherapy treatments. I've already been on the Lahey Clinic website a few times, searching for as much information as possible about my doctors. I've even seen his photograph and thought he was in his forties. However, the man standing in front of us now, hand extended in welcome, is nowhere near forty. He looks like he just graduated yesterday from college, not to mention medical school. Jeff and I shake his hand in turn as he introduces himself. He is tall with curly black hair and a fine square jaw; his handshake is warm and strong, but I feel guarded now as I'm worried that he might be too young.

He pulls up a chair from a corner of the room and asks me what my understanding is of what has happened and what is going to happen. I'm thinking that never in my life have I heard a man's voice as deep as his, and I'm also thinking that he can't possibly be experienced enough to know what he's doing. I want to stick my head out the door and call for another doctor. But I don't do that. I briefly touch the necklace roped on my wrist and reassure myself that if I'm not comfortable with any of these doctors I will ask for a different one.

I clear my throat, wondering if he asks this question of all his patients when he first meets them. Is it a test of some sort, to see how intelligent a response he will get, to see exactly what kind of a person he'll be working with? Because certainly, *he* knows what has already "happened" to me and has a pretty good idea about what is coming next. But he has asked a question and is waiting for my response. Does it really matter if it's a test or not?

I tell him about the calcifications, the biopsy, the surgery, about the not-clear margins and the microscopic cancer cell on one node. I say I understand I'm to have more surgery- a reincision lumpectomy and an axillary node dissection. I see that he is listening carefully while I am talking: he is leaning forward in his chair, and his eyes are on me the whole time. He hasn't brought anything to write with or take notes on, and this makes me feel better as soon as I notice this. There's nothing more exasperating than watching a doctor scribble things in a folder that you can't see while you're talking. I like that he is empty-handed and simply listening, doctor to patient. Putting a notebook and pen between us would only add more boundaries, more formalities.

He says I seem to have a good understanding of the big picture, then proceeds to tell me that I will need to have chemotherapy treatments. He offers me some good news too. If all goes well with the surgery, I'll be able to take part in a Clinical Trial which features a fairly new drug called taxotere.

When he invites my questions, I ask him how long it takes for a precancerous cell to become cancerous. He pauses for a moment, then tells me he really doesn't know. It seems that there are all kinds of factors involved in that answer, and he goes on to explain some of those factors but I'm not absorbing any of it. I do feel greatly satisfied that I have a doctor who can say *I don't know* when he needs to, instead of trying to sound superior with medical double talk and mumbo jumbo.

I muse on this for a while after he leaves, until Dr. Karp knocks and enters. I feel totally glad and reassured to see him. Has it really only been four weeks since I met him? He pulls up the chair that Dr. Morganstern just left, straddles it, and begins talking with us like we were in mid-conversation. He has a bright red plastic folder containing information on the Clinical Trial that I am now eligible for. He talks to us about the importance of research, about Lahey Clinic's involvement with research and clinical trials. Some of this information is way over my head and I happily tune it out. On second thought, perhaps it isn't over my head, just out of range of what I can possibly absorb right now.

He is talking now about the three drugs in the trial- adriamycin, cytoxin and taxotere. The point of the study is to see how taxotere works separately from and in addition to the other two standard chemotherapy drugs. At one point I ask him about the effectiveness of taxotere as I have not heard of it in all my internet research. He loves questions like this, I can tell. They bring out the scientist/researcher in him which I can see is a big part of his love of medicine. He talks for several minutes about trials involving taxotere in Canada and in the States, and while he is spouting these statistics, my already overwhelmed brain is shutting down.

However, I do hear him very clearly when he tells us that if his 43 year old wife was diagnosed with breast cancer, he'd make sure..... no, he'd *insist* that she get taxotere as well as the other drugs. Yes, this is a piece of information that makes its way through my entire body, mind, and soul. I relax into this new bit of knowledge. If taxotere is good enough for my breast surgeon's wife, then it surely is good enough for me. Bring it on.

Dr. Karp also stays with us for a good half hour. I have more questions for him about the upcoming surgery. He answers all of them patiently. I have the feeling (with him also) that if I needed him to sit here for two more hours, he would gladly do it and not once look at his watch.

My last question is the same one I just asked my oncologist: how long does it take a precancerous cell to become cancerous? I believed Dr. Morganstern but I'm curious now to hear what Dr. Karp will say. Will he agree with Dr. Morganstern? Will he try to act like he really knows the answer when there obviously isn't one? Or what if there is a real answer and Dr. Morganstern didn't know it? This surely is my own little investigation into the minds of these two doctors to whom I'm entrusting my life.

He doesn't come right out and say *I don't know*, but he does say that it's hard to tell because there are so many underlying factors. In essence, it's the same answer and I'm happy with it, even though there is no answer. I'm thinking now that some women would probably be distressed by the knowledge that there are precancerous cells inside of them and no one knows if they're turning into cancer cells right at this moment. However, I find that I can't be upset about it. Both doctors have reassured me that the chemotherapy treatments will take care of any cancer cells in my body (pre- or otherwise) and I am choosing to believe that they are right.

Pam, the social worker, comes in next. She is tall with a strong, vibrant face, dark eyes, and beautiful thick black hair. She's wearing a deep emerald green jacket and I pause to admire it after she comments on the turquoise sweater lying beside me. She talks about the Support Group that begins next month. She also tells us about various wig shops in the area that have been recommended by other patients. She tells me how I can use her as a resource, then gives me her phone number and says she's often not at her desk but she'll get right back to me if I leave a message. I believe her immediately. I can tell she's the kind of person who follows through on her promises. When she gets up to leave, I nod towards the examining table and jokingly ask her if she's sure she doesn't want to examine me also. She hesitates, then sees my grin and the twinkle in my eye, and laughs with me.

I know that there is nothing funny about breast cancer, but I'm determined to remain light in spirit anyway. It makes me thoroughly happy right down to my soul when I can make others laugh as their paths touch mine on this strange, unexpected journey.

My Radiation Oncologist knocks on the door a few minutes after Pam leaves. I have to chuckle at all of the knocking going on here today. On the one hand, of course, it is extraordinarily polite. On the other hand, what do they think they might be interrupting? Do they think that Jeff and I have suddenly begun making out on the sterile silver examining table? Do they think we may be taking a nap?

Dr. Girshovich is a tall, solidly built woman with a kind smile and soft wavy brown hair. I'm startled to notice that she's *not* wearing a doctor's jacket, just a soft flowing blue and brown dress that flatters her figure and hair. Her Russian accent is strong and lyrical. She tells me that my radiation treatments won't be until after the chemo is finished. She calls me a *young, strong, healthy voman* and says that I will do well with all of the treatments. This makes me feel especially good (especially the *young* part!) and I find it easy to relax in her presence.

Tuesday January 15

I am driving to Lahey in Burlington for a bone scan which will tell us whether or not the cancer has spread to my bones. This is such a grueling, terrifying image (cancer, eating away my once solid bones) that I determine not to think about it, because what good will it do me really? I'm pretty sure it probably hasn't spread anywhere yet, but... Well, that *but* is terrifying and I don't want it to ruin my day.

In the lobby, I stop at the information desk and hand the receptionist a large brown envelope with Dr. Karp's name and office number on it. Inside is a handmade collage calendar I've made for his office. I've also written a short letter expressing how much I appreciate his care and expertise, and how very well taken care of I feel at this hospital. The receptionist promises that it will be delivered today, and I go on my way feeling much lighter, happier. The act of giving has always had the power to make me feel happy; I'm glad that I have acknowledged and honored this sacred aspect of myself.

After wandering down a few wrong corridors, I find the right office. The nurse takes me into a small room and gives me a big glass of something to drink. She tells me to drink three or four more big glasses of water in the next two hours, and then to come back. She is explaining everything in medical terminology but I tune her out and imagine this strange liquid lighting up my bones so that the scan will be possible.

I spend the two hours in the hospital cafeteria, sipping hot decaf and drinking my water. I have chosen a table next to the wide windows and am looking out on a dreary gray sky.

Well, I think, here I am. It's only been a month and four days since my diagnosis, and my whole world has been tilted on its once very strong axis. But it's still me sitting here, still me wearing this forest green chenille sweater and blue jeans. Still me, curly brown hair, green eyes and glasses, silver swan ring on my right hand, wedding and engagement rings on my left. All the identifying features are the same, so it's still me. Isn't it?

I feel so different inside, like some major spring cleaning has been going on in my mind and spirit. A college friend used to liken this feeling of inner transformation to angels moving the furniture around within our souls, and I've never so clearly understood the meaning of this until right this minute. The angels are definitely doing some interior redecorating; I can feel the subtle changes within me daily.

There are outside changes as well, but they are happening more slowly: a scar below my armpit, a small scar on my lower left breast, the angry black and blue stain covering my right hand from where an IV needle ripped out. And I'm aware that there are more physical changes to come: bigger scars, hair loss, dry skin…. to name a few.

One of the interior changes I've noticed has made itself very clear to me today. I've been watching myself navigate my way around this hospital with confidence bordering on joy. I find this absolutely amazing. Hospitals were once foreign territory to me, scary and intimidating. My only experience with hospitals up until now has been visits to my father and grandmother, before they died. But now the word *hospital* invokes a welcoming familiarity. I find myself anticipating whatever is next, looking forward to the next interesting person I'm going to meet on this strange yet wondrous journey I've been called to.

Why am I not dreading this next surgery? Perhaps I'm enjoying the extra attention. I do like being here, as close to the healers as I can get. Or perhaps it's a survival mechanism- if I open and give voice to the endless possible negative outcomes, I will surely self-destruct within seconds. So maybe it's a choice that I make. When I first found out I had to have another surgery, I was devastated, angry, betrayed, full of grief. But now I've shifted my thinking about the whole situation. I can feel angry and depressed and resistant OR I can say to myself *Well, let's look at what could possibly be good about this.* And I am choosing the latter. This choice brings me immense comfort, peace, relief.

Of course, I don't know for certain that this cancer isn't going to kill me. I don't *think* that it will. I hope and pray that it *won't*. I haven't asked Dr. Karp if it's going to kill me because I don't think this is a fair question to ask (yet) and I know that the answer is dependent on many different things. He has already told me (without my having to ask) that the prognosis for Stages 1-3 is very, very good. He also said if he found more than 10 positive lymph nodes, it would be very, very bad. I'm thinking that if there's a *correct* answer, it's God who knows it, not Dr. Karp.

Finally, after numerous glasses of water and trips to the bathroom, it's time to go back upstairs. The bone scan is painless. I lie on my back in a quiet white room and the table I'm on moves slowly while the machinery overhead scans my body. Amazing to think that this machine can penetrate right through to the innermost parts of my skeleton. I close my eyes while the table moves imperceptibly slowly. The technician says it will take half an hour and that I must lie very still or they might have to do the scan again. No problem. I start some very slow and deep rhythmic breathing.

She continues to chat with me about her son's soccer team and the fundraiser they're having this weekend and whether she should make potato salad or macaroni salad. I keep my eyes closed as I listen to her. Although I don't reply, it gives me great comfort to be reminded that there is a real world out there, outside of this hospital, these tests, my disease. A real world where little boys play soccer, and mothers worry about what to make for fundraising suppers.

Back at the theatre, the afternoon goes more quickly. I dive right in to the piles of subscription renewals, soon engrossed in this unique game of musical chairs (no pun intended), only slightly aware of the people around me, the chatter in the room, the cloudy cold sky outside my window.

My phone rings and I answer it, frowning at the sudden distraction. It's Dr. Karp and he's telling me there's been a surgery cancellation for this

Thursday, so would I like to have my surgery then? *Thursday?* The day after *tomorrow?* I try to remain calm, cool, and collected, but he must hear the panic in my voice. He says he knows it's very short notice but he wanted to see if I'd like to do it earlier and get it over with. I tell him I will think about it and call him back in a few hours.

I do think about it. What else *can* I think about, really? I talk it over with Jeff, then with Suzanne and John at the office. They all tell me to go ahead and do it now. "The sooner the better" used to be an old cliché but today it has new meaning for me. I call Dr. Karp back and tell him yes.

CHAPTER NINE

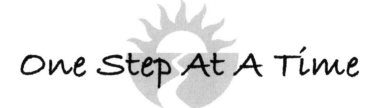

One Step At A Time

Courage is not the absence of fear, but rather the judgment
that something else is more important than fear.
— Ambrose Redmoon

Thursday January 17

I'm sitting at the computer in Jeff's study, staring out the open window at this bright and windy day. The air is rather warm for a New England winter morning. The peace candle glows and fills the room with the subtle fragrance of vanilla. I'm waiting for Jeff's sister Jan to pick me up and drive me to the hospital for my second surgery.

I've been thinking about courage a lot lately. Several people have commented on how courageously I'm handling all of this. One friend even ended her email with *I admire your courage*. Another friend told me she admires me because I'm not responding to the cancer like a victim. All of this is interesting feedback. But I wonder….. am I really that courageous? It's not like I've chosen any of this. I have a microscopic cancerous tumor on one of my lymph nodes, and there are precancer cells inside my left breast. This surgery is not optional.

I've read that courage is feeling the fear and doing it anyway. Well, that's true. I am definitely feeling the fear but I'm having the surgery anyway.

And what am I afraid of exactly? Not waking up from the anesthesia, for one thing. For another thing, the pain I most likely will feel afterwards. Also, the results of the pathology report. How many lymph nodes are positive for cancer? I'm hoping, praying, that none of them are. Less than four would be the next best alternative. But I can't control any of these results. I can only take one step at a time, put one foot in front of me, and then the other, and on and on. This is the only way I can continue the journey.

So then, is courage something I can consciously choose? I wake up, I shower, I dress, I decide to be courageous today and go to surgery? No, I don't think that's how it is. The courage lives somewhere deep inside of me, in every one of us. It just takes different situations to activate it.

What I consciously choose is to accept the fear, to take deep breaths and remain centered no matter what happens, to scan my thoughts continually in order to transform any negativity lurking there into thoughts of a more positive nature.

A few days ago I was able to slow down enough to actually hear these pessimistic thoughts. *Oh dear God, I don't want to have another surgery. This is awful. There is more cancer inside of me. This is so much worse than I thought.*

But because I was able to identify them as destructive, I was able to replace them with some more hopeful thoughts: *Thank God my doctor took out two nodes instead of just the first one. The tumor is microscopic; I'm glad it's not full-sized. The cells in my breast are precancerous; I'm glad they're not cancerous. It's a good thing we found this early and that I have such a good doctor. And besides all that, I get to have an extra week off from work!*

I don't know if changing my thinking patterns takes courage. Maybe it does. But I do know it's healthier for me. I do know that I feel better physically and emotionally when I do it. It's like choosing what to eat based on how you'll feel afterwards, rather than the taste of it right now.

The chemo has been on my mind a lot lately, too. I'll be starting those treatments in a few weeks, and then another few weeks after that, my hair will begin falling out. So I need to get a wig. I've been consciously working on changing my thought patterns around this subject as well. These are the thoughts that have been going round and round in my mind about the chemo and the hair loss: *But I really, really like my hair and want to keep it. It's going to be so annoying to have to put on a wig every morning. What if it's scratchy and hot? I don't want people feeling sorry for me when they find out I've lost my hair. What if it blows away and everyone sees my bald head?*

So whenever I hear one of those panic-ridden, negative thoughts, I notice and acknowledge it, then choose to replace it with a different thought. Here are the ones I've come up with so far. *Hey, this will be my chance to try out another hairstyle. No more bad hair days. Look at the time I'll save not having to wash and condition and dry my hair every morning. Think of the money I'll save not having to buy conditioners and hair coloring every month.*

I'm sure that when the time comes, I'll have some tears about this, but I'm not going to cry about it just yet. I'm going to take one breath at a time and see if I can get myself through this surgery first.

My journaling has absorbed me so deeply that Jan is ringing the doorbell before I know it. I grab my tote bag into which I've stuffed my new teddy bear. I've draped a bright pink ribbon around her neck as well as my favorite necklace from Kripalu. I want her to be the first thing I see when I wake up. Also in the tote bag is my toothbrush, some sinus medicine, lip moisturizer, another new cotton front closure bra one size too big, and a clean pair of underwear. I'm wearing my gray cotton yoga pants and a man's XXL soft corduroy shirt (no more pullover sweaters for me for a while) in a deep shade of turquoise that makes me happy just looking at it.

I was right about Jan. She is calm and attentive; being near her is just what I need. She maintains just the right level of distraction. We talk about her upcoming trip to France; we talk about my niece Stephanie who is spending this semester in Paris. In the waiting room we flip through decorating magazines together, admiring the photographs. For a few moments I'm fooled into thinking I'm in the dentist's office waiting for a routine cleaning.

In about half an hour, a nurse calls my name and all images of the dentist's waiting room quickly disappear. Jan hugs me goodbye and I give my coat to the nurse, stuffing my new scarf into the tote bag so it is draped around the teddy bear. The scarf is from my friend Sue, and is hand knit in the most beautiful shades of fuchsia and purple. The colors themselves warm me from the inside out and I want them to be visible when I'm emerging from the anesthetic haze.

I take off every last article of clothing and put them in the bright yellow plastic bag lying on the bed. Then I put on the thin hospital gown, a light grayish blue with little red and black geometrical designs, tied in the back. This is all so surreal. Wasn't I just here, doing the exact same thing, thinking it would be the one and only time?

After sitting on the edge of the bed for fifteen minutes, I'm tired of waiting for someone to attend to me so I lie down and pull the stiff gray blanket around me for warmth. I lie very still, listening to the mellow sound of my breath, which relaxes and comforts me.

It's quiet here today, unlike the hustle and bustle of organized chaos that was happening last time. Across the hall I can see a thin elderly man and his wife who is fussing over him. Every few minutes a doctor or nurse walks by, their pace measured and graceful. I admire their freedom to be up and about, business as usual. This is my business today: lying here, waiting for the healing to begin.

Finally, the nurse peers in and cheerfully says she hasn't forgotten me and is coming right back. The anesthesiologist comes in and I'm happy to see it's the same one, plain blue cap and all. He still seems young but not as young as I remembered him. Genuinely nice, compassionate, kind. He asks if I know why I'm here and once again I'm struck with the absurdity of this question. Does *any* woman lying in a presurgical bed awaiting a second lumpectomy *not* know the answer to this question? I find myself showing off a bit, using words like *axillary* and *re-excision*. He nods, listening carefully, then tells me he's going to try to find the paperwork from last time so he doesn't have to ask me the same medical history questions again. He disappears around the corner with a little wave, and I am alone again.

I tell myself to relax, and bring my focus back to my breath. I find that I'm fairly sleepy.

I feel ready. Lifted. Held.

Dr. Karp comes in and tells me they're running a little behind in the O.R. He still has one more patient before me and it'll probably be an hour and a half before they wheel me in. I tell him not to worry, I'm not going anywhere, and he laughs. I like the sound of this. He moves to the right side of my bed and tells me that he absolutely loves the calendar I made for him. He says he just can't get over how beautiful my collages are, and that now he has *real art* hanging in his office. I wonder if he knows this is the highest compliment he could give me. I am touched and pleased, although I'm still wondering if I've crossed some invisible doctor-patient boundary by giving him a gift. I've read many books on breast cancer, but not one of them has addressed the issue of giving a gift to your doctor.

At 3:15 they finally wheel me into the O.R. The first thing I see is Dr. Karp sitting in the back left corner of the room on a stool. I keep my eyes on him while I go through the undignified process of being shifted from the bed-on-wheels to the surgical table. This leaves me feeling somewhat powerless and humiliated, yet I am comforted by the surprising tenderness in his eyes. I wonder why he is simply sitting in the corner. Then I realize that his role as surgeon doesn't involve this part of the process; he is simply waiting in the wings for his cue to come onstage.

After they have me centered on the narrow metal table, he comes over to my left side and I see another look of tenderness. Not pity, not detached professionalism, not joviality. All of these things are what I might have expected were I not on this journey. But it is tenderness I see in my doctor's eyes today and I let it wash over me like soft rain on a hot afternoon.

The anesthesiologist stretches both of my arms out onto the side metal tables which weren't there last time. I know they are readying my left arm for the lymph node dissection, but I wonder why my other arm is also stretched out. They cover my right arm with a towel and I'm immediately grateful because it's freezing in here and now my right side at least is warm.

This crucifixion pose leaves me feeling incredibly vulnerable. Dr. Karp is still beside me and now he is massaging my left arm. His hands are warm and the gentle stroking and pulling of the muscles and skin feels welcome and soothing. I know he's prepping my arm, getting the blood moving for the surgery, but I relax into his confident touch and close my eyes. I'm no longer scared and anxious, just relieved that he is here with his brightly colored surgical cap, relieved that he knows me, that I feel cared about and cared for, glad that this whole thing is almost over.

Then the oxygen mask is placed over my nose and that's it. No prolonged plunging into the dark realms of sleep, no endless dreams, no visions, no nightmares…. Only seconds of darkness and it feels like I am starting to come awake.

I can tell I'm still in the O.R. by the sounds around me. A man's voice is asking me if I can hear him, but I don't recognize his voice. I feel stiff and inert but find myself nodding my head ever-so-slightly.

Soon there are more voices around me, and I wonder why there are so many people. My eyelids feel like they are glued to my eyeballs and my head is aching now too. Some of the voices are urging me to lean over to the right so they can slip a board under me which will enable them to lift me onto the gurney. Surely this is impossible, I'm thinking, but I manage to do what I'm told, and they lift me carefully onto the stretcher. In the midst of this, I hear a woman's voice asking who she should call if…..

If what, I wonder, helpless, frantic.

But I immediately relax into the familiar cadence of Dr. Karp's voice, telling her to call *him* if anything should happen. It's fine then, I'm thinking. Everything will be okay if he's still here.

Now I'm being wheeled down a long corridor, then bumpety-bump into an elevator, feeling the motion of going quickly down, down, down. Then bumpety-bump out and down a few more corridors. I feel dizzy, afraid to open my eyes which are feeling not quite as heavy now. They ask me to lean over to the right again so they can lift me off the gurney and onto the hospital bed. I'm still in a mighty haze but am able to open my eyes and focus for a few seconds. I see Jeff standing beside the bed and an instant smile graces my lips. He points to the foot of my bed where he's propped up my teddy bear. I giggle a little to see her there wearing the bright scarf and my special necklace, then close my eyes against my will and drift off to sleep, still feeling heavy, warm, stiff, immobile.

When I open my eyes next, Jeff is sitting in the chair beside my bed and there's a nurse standing beside me, talking with him in a very low voice. Her name is Jan and she is tall with short, light wavy hair. Having her near me feels entirely cooling and calming.

Jeff feeds me ice chips when I ask for them, or rubs them on my lips. I'm still feeling drugged and borderline nauseous. I feel the need to take deep, deep breaths, but my breathing is very shallow, almost to the point of nonexistence. I don't think I've ever breathed this shallowly before; it's almost as if I might stop breathing altogether.

I feel an almost excruciating need to be touched, so I ask Jeff to lay his hands on my head, my forehead, my neck, my shoulders. This simple touch feels unbelievably good and he continues to do this for several minutes.

I doze off for a while and when I awaken at 7:00, I realize I have to go to the bathroom. It takes a while to dawn on me that this is not going to be as simple as it sounds. Jan comes in and she is patient, telling me which part of my body to move first, and where, and how. She moves the IV beside me as we walk in slow motion to the bathroom which is a mere ten feet from the bed. It feels like the longest walk of my life.

At 11:00 I hear more noise in the hallway at the nurse's station which is across from my room. It seems far away because my door is shut, but I can hear the sounds of laughter and conversation as the nurses change shifts. The noise is comforting. It reminds me of how I felt when I was a little girl, going to bed while the grownups were still up and about in the house. Safe and comforted, part of something bigger than myself.

Friday January 18

I sleep until 3 a.m. when I need to go to the bathroom again. It's a little easier this time, but I still need assistance. When I'm settled back in the bed, I lie very still, embracing the silence. This is the first time I'm truly "awake" since before the surgery, and I feel incredibly, sublimely peaceful. The night surrounding me is absolutely quiet. There is nothing for me to do but watch the clock on the wall on the other side of the room. Time moves very slowly in the middle of the night.

There's a painting of a peaceful ocean scene under the clock and it holds my gaze as well. The sea has mesmerized me since I was a child, so just looking at this picture makes me happy, makes me feel just a little bit more like I am home instead of in a hospital. I feel the immediate and comforting presence of Spirit- nothing big or mighty, just a slightly tangible closeness to a loving presence that remains near me, surrounding me with a sense of safety and love. Perhaps it is an angel, or Jesus, or my father coming back for a visit to comfort me. I realize that it doesn't matter what I name it, it simply *is*, and this is simply enough.

I lie completely still, not wanting to move, allowing the serene presence to wash over me like waves caressing the shore. I long to take this stillness, this presence, this feeling, home with me. Is there some way to capture it so I can access it again and again? I drift back to sleep on the wings of this peace.

In a little while, I once again hear the sounds of the nurses changing shifts. The light changes in the hallway and beyond the long vertical blinds.

I turn on the TV and watch the news and weather. I'm lying very still, breathing more normally now but not as fully as I'm used to.

An older woman with tightly curled hair comes in and reads me my choices for breakfast. I manage to eat every bite of the scrambled eggs and English muffin. The urge to use the bathroom strikes full force again, and this time I can do it on my own which gives me a surprising feeling of accomplishment and pride.

Dr. Karp comes in at 8:30, lays his hand on my feet, then reaches over the bed and lifts the cover off the breakfast tray to see what I've eaten. He grins when he sees the empty plate, then asks me how I am.

Oh sure, I think. As if there's a good answer to *that* question the morning after this kind of surgery. I tell him that other than feeling like I've just been run over by a Mack truck, I'm feeling just fine.

He laughs, but I'm thinking he's probably heard that one before. Or maybe not. Maybe other women don't feel like making jokes the morning after this kind of surgery.

He tells me about the drain that's been inserted in a small hole in my left side under my armpit. He shows me how to unhook it, how to empty the fluid twice a day, how to record the number of milliliters that drain each time. He tells me that in the course of the week, the color of the draining fluid will change from merlot to zinfandel. I love this visual analogy; it makes me smile.

He also tells me that the pathology report will be ready next week, probably on Thursday. I somehow find the words to ask if he will call me and he says yes, asking if I will be at home. I tell him not to worry, I'm not going anywhere. He laughs again and the sound brings a clear energy into the room, into my spirit.

My new nurse, Jody, changes my dressings and also shows me how to empty the drain. She helps me into my bra (a bit tricky because of the heavy gauze padding which seems to be everywhere), then leaves Jeff to help me with the rest of my clothes.

On the ride home, I'm entranced with all of it: the bare tree limbs, the cars at the mall, the pale blue winter sky streaked with delicate white clouds. I am entranced, and I am grateful. Grateful to be alive, to be on the road to wellness, to have my husband beside me. Grateful to be going home where a soft bed and my cats await me.

Once home and propped up amongst pillows and sweet-smelling sheets, I expect to be ready for a nap, but find myself wide awake. The sunlight is pouring through the windows, Sasha nestles herself against my hip, and I am once again resting in the precious stillness of Spirit that came to me in the night. I lie motionless, acutely aware of every single thing around me. I am intensely quiet... listening... feeling... rejoicing.

Later this afternoon, I pull out a book of meditations for women living with breast cancer and come across an entry that describes a hospital as a transitional space between our comfortable homes and the medical expertise of healing. The author talks about how a hospital can treat us with "equal doses of technology and tenderness."

I gasp with delight at these words. This is exactly what my surgery experiences have been like, and this is exactly why I admire Dr. Karp so much. He has understood the need for both the technical and the tender aspects of his job, and he has integrated both into his relationships with his patients. If he was too tender, too caring, too sympathetic, it would surely make me cry every time he comes near me. If he was too technical, too aloof, I would surely feel alone and scared. But somehow he knows just the right measure of each. This is the delight. This is the blessing.

Sunday January 19

My whole being still feels slow and quiet. The drain is not as hard to maintain as I thought it would be, but taking a shower turns out to be terribly difficult. My left arm feels heavy and stiff. It hurts to lift it higher than an inch but I'm determined to do this one normal thing. Jeff helps me take off my nightgown, and I step into the shower. My right arm works just fine and I find I can soap myself and wash my hair with my right hand as the drain dangles freely from my left side. The warm water feels incredibly good on my face and body.

When I step out of the shower, I immediately realize that I need Jeff to help me dry off. I can't reach behind me to dry myself, and I can't put the bra on alone either, even if it is a front closure bra that's one size too big. I begin to weep with frustration, so Jeff puts his arms around me in the steamy room, smoothes my wet hair back from my face, and tells me not to worry about it, that he doesn't mind helping me at all.

I'm truly grateful for his steadfast willingness to do what needs to be done, but I'm still feeling a certain loss of dignity, a slight humiliation in the fact that I can't do everything for myself anymore. I know it won't last. I know that I will heal, that the drain will be taken out, that my arm won't always feel this heavy and numb. But right now, in this moment, I cry for my sudden loss of independence.

Eventually I'm dry, the dressings are changed, the bra is back on, and the drain is pinned to the XXL blue plaid shirt that I'm wearing over my gray yoga pants. Men's button-up shirts are much easier to wear than my usual pullover sweaters and tops. I sink back into the bed, exhausted from the effort of this one simple shower.

When Jeff leaves to do some errands, I don't feel like reading and I'm too tired to sit at the computer, so I turn on the TV, flip some channels and settle on *The Princess Diaries,* watching with detached interest.

Towards the end of the movie, the "princess" is reading a letter from her deceased father. I hear the entire letter but there is one sentence that sounds louder and clearer than the others: *Courage is not the absence of fear, but rather the judgment that something else is more important than fear.*

Yes!! Yes!! That is exactly it. I've been trying to define what courage has to do with my breast cancer journey. Trying to make sense of people telling me how courageous I am and how I don't think of it as courage yet somehow it must be.

I understand it now. Family and friends see me expressing courage because I experience the fear, but then I decide that something else (joy, laughter, health) is more important. So it's a choice I make. It's always a choice.

But here's another side of this issue that I find distressing: Mom telling me this morning on the phone how tough and strong I am. Everyone says these things about me and I feel good about it, glad that this is their perception of me. But then when I feel depressed and miserable, I feel guilty. I start thinking they wouldn't be calling me strong, tough and courageous if they could see me sobbing uncontrollably on Jeff's shoulder because I can't even dry myself after a shower.

And yet….. and yet….. of course I'm still courageous. Having courage doesn't entail a complete emotional shut-down. Sometimes it takes plenty of courage and strength just to give in to the tears.

CHAPTER TEN

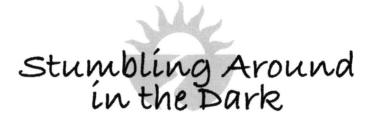

Stumbling Around in the Dark

Our greatest glory is not in never falling,
But in rising every time we fall.

— *Confucius*

Sunday January 20

I'm feeling lonely, pummeled by clouds of dark anger; the winds of change are stirring up more emotion than I have strength for at the moment. It seems like all I've been doing is lying in bed and watching *I Love Lucy* and *Leave It To Beaver* reruns alternately with old Tom Cruise movies. Oh, and did I mention… napping? I feel imprisoned in this bedroom. I'm sure I could be hanging out on the family room sofa downstairs and no one would mind, but there's no way to make that space dark enough for me to sleep. There's no way to make that space inaccessible to anyone who walks in the front door.

This freewheeling anger has to do with the "why me?" syndrome, which I was thinking had passed me by. I see now it has not passed me by at all, it's simply been waiting in the wings for an appropriate string of idle moments to move in and settle down. These *why me* thoughts are swirling around in my head like some crazy tornado, stirring up the angry clouds of self-righteousness.

Jeff is being very good about my temporary invalid status, but he just doesn't *get* what is happening to me. As he was leaving this morning, he grasped my left arm and pulled me to him in a kiss. My *left* arm, three days out of surgery. My *left* arm, which feels like it's been run over by a bulldozer. My *left* arm, my "surgical" arm as the books refer to it. I shrieked in pain; he pulled away quickly, embarrassed that he had forgotten. And then I cried warm tears of guilt for having to push him away.

I feel disabled and imprisoned by the newly heavy weight of my left arm. Will it ever feel "normal" again?

Monday January 21

Four days out of surgery and it is still extremely uncomfortable to move my arm. I'm not exactly in pain and I haven't taken any of the prescription painkillers I was given. The extra-strength Tylenol has been enough. And yet, it feels like there's a bowling ball under my armpit. My arm isn't swollen; I know this for a fact because I check in the mirror every chance I get.

There's only one position I can sleep in and that is flat on my back. The drain and its constant maintenance is becoming more and more annoying as the week goes by, however there is much less liquid now than there was four days ago, and the color is much lighter, leaning closely towards the lighter pink of the zinfandel and away from the darker tones of the merlot. I smile as I remember Dr. Karp's metaphor.

People are continually asking if I'm in pain and I continue to tell them no. What I'm feeling is cloudier than pain, harder to describe. I feel full to the brim of discomfort, like there are lead weights lying heavy on my arm, my mind, my spirit.

And now I have this whole week ahead of me. What I *want* to be doing is playing at my art table, creating some new note card designs. But I cannot do any of this, not this week. I feel handicapped. Handicapped and frustrated. The use of my left arm and entire body is limited right now. I need to rest, lie still, exercise my wrist and fingers. My writing is limited unless I use the computer and even then I can only manage a few minutes at a time before I need to put my arm up on the pillows again.

Tuesday January 22

I'm bored out of my mind, which feels totally ridiculous. A few months ago, I know I would've given *anything* to have all this time on my hands. An entire ten days to myself. I'm about halfway through those ten days now and the worst of the boredom is bearing down on me, hard. I'm feeling lonely and sorry for myself, but I have been allowing myself to cry when the feelings have gotten too deep for anything but tears.

Jeff calls at noon and tells me he has to work a few hours later tonight, and I have to hold the phone away from me for a minute while I try to find my composure. The rational part of me doesn't mind that he's working late. Every once in a while he does. But it seems that this morning I'm not exactly in my rational mind. I am in my loneliness. To be alone, truly alone all day, and then to have to be alone yet a while longer tonight….. I feel completely miserable about this, but I pretend that I'm my usual rational self and tell him it's okay. I'm so tired of asking things of him. I'm so tired of needing him to do everything for me. This at least is something I can do for *him*.

Later, Dr. Karp calls me with good news. The pathology report is back and all nineteen lymph nodes are clear, AND the lumpectomy resulted in clean margins this time! Oh, what sweet relief. No more surgery. No more hospital visits. Just on with the wig purchase. On with the chemo and radiation.

Wednesday January 23

Suzanne calls to ask about my schedule for next week. She asks how I'm feeling and I tell her I'm doing better. No one else has called me, but I've received a ton of emails and cards from friends and family and people at the theatre. I wonder if they're all afraid of disturbing me, waking me up from a nap. I decide to take matters into my own hands and call Joan and John at work this afternoon. It is so blessedly good to hear their voices. I feel a little more human again, a little more connected, a little more alive.

Sleeping tonight is extremely difficult. It seems the after-effects of the anesthesia have finally worn off. I'm extremely uncomfortable in spite of the Tylenol. The bed feels crowded, and Jeff's snoring is out of control. I'm so frustrated that it spills out into tears. I pull on my heavy fleece robe and go to my Quiet Room, sink into my favorite chair by the window, rocking and weeping. Jeff hasn't heard me and I don't want to wake him. What would be the point? He would just pat me on the back and tell me it'll all be over soon, which is how he is dealing with all of this. He would hold me as long as I needed to be held, but it's rather hard to hold me these days because of this damned drain which is in the way, and my damned arm which now feels like hot pins and needles are sticking into it on the back upper side.

I feel so helpless like this, in the middle of the night, so lonely and empty. But I allow myself the feelings. I allow myself the tears. They can't last forever, can they?

Thursday January 24

I wake up feeling groggy and stiff, my arm a solid lead weight at my side. The air feels surprisingly like spring although the sky is still pale gray and the sunlight doesn't seem serious. I use my right hand to open a few windows, then put on sweatpants and an oversized man's shirt over my nightgown. I stand on the front porch for a moment and breathe in the fresh air. It's been an entire week since I've stepped out of the house, so this new freedom feels delightfully delicious to me. I go to the bank, to the corner cafe for some chai, and to the grocery store for ingredients for dinner.

These errands take only thirty minutes, but I'm completely exhausted, so I climb back into bed and sit for a long time in the silence, first with my journal, then with a new novel.

Friday January 25

This morning I put on "real" clothes (jeans, socks, shoes, earrings) for the first time in a week. Jeff is going to drive me to my appointment with Dr. Karp to have the drain removed. This lends an atmosphere of sweet normalcy to the day. My spirits are brightened considerably, just from these few simple things.

As Dr. Karp is washing his hands before he examines me, I somehow manage to keep a straight face while I tell him I've sort of grown accustomed to the drain and have decided to leave it in.

He pauses for one slight beat, then grins and tells me he can't really do that but he'd be happy to let me take it home with me if I'd like it for a souvenir.

I chuckle as I lie back on the table. Excellent comeback. He reminds me to breathe deeply and tells me it might hurt a little, but before I can even process this, he's holding the drainage bulb up beside me, free and clear. He covers the opening under my armpit with a gauze bandage, then tells me to get dressed and disappears around the sliding oak door.

When he comes back, he talks about the chemo treatments, and answers all of our questions patiently. He tells me to think of him as the quarterback of my team, that he is the coordinator of my care, the one calling the plays, and not to hesitate to call him with any questions, anytime. This metaphor means more to Jeff than it does to me, although I do have a vague sense of the importance of the quarterback to a football team. Jeff suggests that maybe I could think of Dr. Karp as an orchestra conductor instead, since that is a more artistic image in tune with (no pun intended) my life at the theatre. I leave his office once again feeling uplifted, safe, secure.

After lunch, my brother Joe brings Mom for a visit. It does me a world of good to see them, to be hugged by them. However, the look of pity in Mom's eyes is still hard to bear. What I've been through has been difficult, yes, but I've been so well taken care of through it all that I don't feel it's necessary for people to feel sorry for me. We sit in the family room, talking. Sasha curls up on my lap and I'm calmed immediately by the simple warm weight of her body.

Joe has brought me several books of humorous stories and cartoons. He's also brought me Norman Cousins' book *Anatomy of an Illness*, which is about how he healed himself from a rare blood disease with massive doses of Vitamin C and laughter. I receive the book with surprise and gladness. I first read this book about fifteen years ago, using it as a starting point for a workshop on the power of humor that I led for the teachers I was working with then. I remember being fascinated with the whole concept of humor's power to heal, and actually incorporated some of that philosophy into my daily life, never knowing at the time that one day the topic would be of life-giving importance to me.

I'm especially touched because not only is Joe giving me the book, he has inscribed it especially for me, and he has read it himself, making notes on certain pages and pointing out certain facts that resonated with him. This book is pure gift in so many ways, and I'm anxious to read it again, this time with a more intimate knowledge of the topic at hand.

Mom has brought several books and pamphlets on healing and "positive thinking." I feel anger and frustration rising in me as she lays the books in front of me. She talks about how she uses the affirmations in one of the booklets every day. The feelings simmer and scald their way through my whole being, reminding me of my adolescence where I was often cornered and lectured on topics that I already knew something about. I breathe my way through these feelings now, remembering that she really does mean well, and I reassure her that I've got a pretty good grasp on the topic of positive thinking. I look into her eyes and the intensity of my feelings diminish considerably. She is genuinely worried about me, I can see that. She knows she can't control what is happening to me, and this is the only thing she can think of that might help.

So I accept Mom's books with a smile, but also with a certain sadness. I wish my mother and I were close enough that she could have asked me about how I'm dealing with all of this first, before giving me these books. To be honest, I'm wishing we were close enough that she would have noticed that I *already am* facing all of this with a positive and open attitude towards healing. Isn't she curious about how I'm approaching this strange new journey? I know she's interested, it's just that she believes there is only one way to experience healing, and because of this, I feel like she's trying to force it on me without even stopping to notice who I am in this moment.

After they leave I take a short nap, then head downtown for a manicure and pedicure. I've always handled stress and tension by biting my fingernails. Since the surgery, I've become aware that bitten nails and cuticles are more open to infection, and any infections in my left hand or arm could mean the onset of lymphedema. This has frightened me into deciding to have a manicure every other week, something I've always wanted to do for myself but never made a priority. I like the feeling of turning my hands and feet over to this young Oriental woman, who smoothes them and fusses over them until they look beautiful. I'm not accustomed to pampering myself but I decide I could definitely get used to it.

At home later, Jeff suggests we go out for Indian food which I dearly love. I don't think I can possibly do one more thing without collapsing from exhaustion, but the lure of my favorite food entices me to go with him. The lamb korma is creamy and spicy, and the coconut Nan is hot and sweet. It feels absolutely delightful to be out in a restaurant like a normal person once again, having dinner side by side with my husband.

Saturday January 26

This morning I drive the mile to the theatre, pick up my paycheck and deposit it in the bank. When I get home, I feel like I've run a marathon. There goes my total energy expenditure for one day. I spend the rest of the day reading in bed, my left arm propped up on two big pillows. I had no idea I was going to be this exhausted, this uncomfortable. I suppose it's all part of the healing process, but it's been more than a week and I'm sick and tired of this damned *healing process*. Indeed, I am weary of it all.

I…JUST…WANT…MY…OLD…LIFE…BACK. My former life… where I could do what I wanted, when I wanted. I remember thinking earlier this week how all this peace and quiet is so good for me, how it's teaching me to slow down, how it's teaching me patience. But after ten days, the peace and quiet really sucks. I've had enough. If I could just go into my Quiet Room and work on a collage, I think I would feel better. But I'm not up to the creative process either. I'm just not up to it.

My depression also stems from the guilt I feel about how drastically our sex life has changed because of my illness, because of my surgery. After the second surgery, I had to ask Jeff to sleep in the armchair for a few nights. I felt guilty about that but I couldn't sleep for fear of him jostling and injuring my left arm. He's being so kind and sweet about the whole thing, but I can't help feeling bad about it. He's back to sleeping in our bed, but a few nights ago I asked if we could switch sides because it was more comfortable for me that way.

Why didn't anyone prepare me for *this* part of the recovery process?

Elizabeth's email is reassuring. She tells me I have earned the right to complain and whine a little. After all I've just had two surgeries in fourteen days, plus I'm facing: chemotherapy, hair loss, radiation, and a radical change in my life patterns and plans. She's right. I'm aware of all of this. I do have the right to grumble and groan. So I allow myself the luxury of this unhappiness for a while. But I refuse to let myself wallow in it much longer than a few hours. I bring some old magazines to the bed and start cutting them up for future collage projects. This makes me smile, reminding me that someday soon I will have enough energy to play at my art table again.

Monday January 28

I'm glad to be back at the theatre among friends, but the work day is tiring, to say the least. By 1:00 I'm ready for my daily nap but I somehow manage to keep my eyes open until 4:00. I was planning to take a nap when I got home but find myself eating popcorn and cookies to comfort myself instead. I feel frustrated at the limitations my body is placing on me. I'm tired of being tired, tired of not being able to make love, tired of everything. Worried that my arm is never going to feel any better. Tired of how it all hurts. Longing for normal.

Also, I feel quite empty inside. There is a deep inexplicable sadness at the core of me when I think of letting go of my position at the theatre. I've already asked for a leave of absence during my treatments. Suzanne told me not to worry, that my job would be there for me when I'm ready to come back. I suggested that John and I switch job titles. He is definitely ready for the increased responsibility, and they have both agreed to this. It feels so right. I'm grateful that John is there for me to turn things over to, that I can leave for several months and feel like the projects I've initiated and shaped for so long will be in good, competent hands.

Saturday February 2

My arm feels surprisingly better and it's easier to move. I can put my arm against my side without feeling like there's a volleyball there, and am pleased with this noticeable measure of improvement.

This afternoon we go out for Mexican food with JoAnn and Jim. We haven't been out with them since before my diagnosis, so this excursion is especially nourishing for me. I revel in the feeling of being almost normal again although I know that chemotherapy lurks around the corner. For today I'm content to put it out of my mind and relax into the company of my husband and good friends.

After lunch we drive to a nearby theatre to see the movie *A Beautiful Mind.* I'm worried (as usual) about my left arm, so we take five seats on an aisle with me sitting the farthest in, my left arm propped up on all of our coats which are resting in the empty seat to my left.

The theatre fills up quickly and soon people are asking if the seat next to me is taken. At first I feel guilty, telling them they can't sit there. But then I think of my sisters on the Survivor's Board, and the guilt melts away. I need that extra seat for my arm. If someone sits there, my arm will have to be positioned into my lap and it will be extremely uncomfortable. The theatre darkens and the previews begin. A few more people ask about the seat; JoAnn whispers to them about my surgery and they go away. I refuse to feel badly for them; if they really wanted a good seat, they should have come earlier!

When I first accepted that I had breast cancer, I promised myself not to apologize to anyone for it, no matter how much it inconvenienced anyone else. Today I choose to take care of myself instead of apologizing. This may seem like a tiny thing on the outside, but inside I feel like I've completed a marathon of psychological growth. Taking care of myself has to be my primary consideration now and I'm learning exactly what that means in the real world.

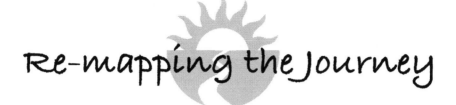

CHAPTER ELEVEN

Re-mapping the Journey

Knowing your destination is only half the journey.

— Anonymous

Sunday February 3

I'm sitting on the bed innocently reading a magazine when the phone rings. And even though I can only hear Jeff's side of the conversation, I know it's Cheryl (his ex) because his voice is raised and he hardly ever raises his voice.

After he hangs up, he sits on the edge of the big green recliner and tells me that Cheryl wants their 16 year old daughter Merri to live with *us* from now on. She wants him to drive an hour to her house on the South Shore and pick Merri up *right now*. He says he told her that he's going to talk it over with me first.

I feel fury akin to fire coursing through my blood, my bones, my mind. How dare they even consider this a possibility? Unlike Jeff, I make no effort to curb my anger. If I keep it in, I will surely self-destruct.

If Merri lives with us now, *I* will be the one responsible for getting her to school every morning, for picking her up every afternoon, for making sure her homework is done, that she is somewhere safe every day after school. Even though I love her very much, this is something I just can't deal with right now.

No, I tell him emphatically. NO. This is simply not an option in our family right now. I've never said no to him regarding anything to do with his children. But I am choosing to say no now.

No. These next five months are for *me*. There is something in my body that can kill me and I need to spend all of my time and energy fighting it. The words fly out of my mouth full of outrage. But as proud as I am of myself for taking care of myself here by saying no, my heart is breaking. As much as Jeff and I have always hoped and dreamed that one day Merri would come to live with us, I have to say no to this for now. This time, I have to put myself first.

I suggest attempting a compromise with Cheryl. Perhaps she and her new husband can keep Merri with them until the end of the school year and then in the summer when my treatments are over, she can move in with us permanently.

I'm fairly hysterical with tears and Jeff holds me while I come back to myself. So many times in our stepfamily, I have been the "bad guy" and now here I am again in this despicable yet familiar role. I'm afraid that my vehemently furious and steadfast *no* is going to drive us far apart, but that doesn't seem to be happening. Here he is, standing beside me, arms around me, and I feel as safe and sheltered as ever.

Several emotional phone calls later, it is determined that Merri will live with Jeff's sister Jan and her family for the rest of the school year. They live three miles from us and it seems like the ideal solution. I silently bless them for stepping in to take care of Merri during this difficult time. If there is any safe and emotionally healthy place for Merri to be right now, it is with them.

Since my diagnosis, I thought that I'd never need to apologize to anyone for having breast cancer. But tonight I tell Jeff many, many times how sorry I am for having to say no. If I didn't have cancer, this wouldn't be an issue. Having Merri come to live with us would simply be a dream come true for us. We've wanted Merri to live with us for so long. But now that it's happening, a magical gift we never expected to be offered, we have to temporarily refuse it. Because of me. I am indeed very sorry. I do indeed apologize. I wish this wasn't happening to me, to us. I wish with all my heart and soul and body that we could say yes, but we can't. I can't. And still, Jeff seems to understand. This fills me with incredible relief and silent joy.

Tuesday February 5

After work today I find that all I have energy for is watching television. The afternoon is dark and I feel a slight depression slithering into my body. I want to be up and about, doing ordinary things like making supper, taking a walk, creating new card designs. But there is no energy left after working all day, and now I'm feeling sad and useless.

When Jeff comes home, he brings me the mail which includes a card from his oldest daughter Amanda. She has written a lovely note telling me she's sorry about my diagnosis and that she wants me to know she's here for me like I was there for her so many years ago. Her words touch me in a deep, new place.

Thursday February 7

I've wanted for some time now to have professional massage on a regular basis but have always put it off, thinking I couldn't afford it. The phrase *there's no moment like the present* floats through my mind and suddenly it's no longer a cliché. I am now having manicures every week, and I remember a time when I didn't think I could afford that either. So I call Lucy, the massage therapist I went to a few years ago, and we schedule an appointment for next week.

Tonight I'm propped up in bed reading when Merri stops by so Jeff can sign some papers for school. Soon I hear light footsteps on the stairs, and suddenly Merri is here, her bright and lovely presence in the doorway. She asks how I am, comes over to my side of the bed and lightly kisses me on the cheek. There are tears in my eyes at the gentle reassurance of her kiss, her touch, her presence. I was afraid she'd be angry with me and think I was rejecting her, but this doesn't appear to be so. We talk for a few minutes about her new school and Aunt Jan's cat (Blue) who might just be related to our Sasha.

I love you, she calls lightly as she leaves the room, and my heart fills with a soft and simple gratitude.

Friday February 8

I go to work today knowing that Monday will be my last day at the theatre for several months. This is a hard fact to get used to, as the theatre has been an integral part of my life for so long. I'm wondering if I really will come back here when my treatments are over. Will I really want to come back? I'm hoping to figure this out over the next several months, hoping somehow to learn what I really want to do next.

Next week Suzanne will be away on business so she won't be here on my last day. This afternoon before she leaves, she comes to my desk and says goodbye, opening her arms to me for a light hug. I am filled with emotion at this display of affection.

I still can't believe this is happening to me- cancer, surgery, chemo, radiation. I really can't believe any of it. I'm doing what I have to do each moment of every day to get myself through it, but most of the time it seems unreal, like I'm watching a play unfold where I'm onstage and in the audience at the same time. Until a moment like this one- my boss hugs me goodbye and we're all acutely aware that it's because I'm leaving for cancer treatments. Suddenly, for an instant, it's very clear that this *is* real, that this most definitely *is* happening to *me*.

Monday February 11

Dr. Morganstern is twenty minutes late for our pre-chemotherapy appointment. He apologizes as soon as he walks in, and my annoyance immediately dissolves. He still seems very young to me, and he doesn't call me by name once during the whole hour. But I do have the sense that he knows exactly what he's talking about and that I'm in good hands, that he is gifted with a clear, calm intelligence, that he won't let me down.

He gives me a brief physical exam, then orders a blood test and an EKG. After these tests, I will need to sit with Mary for a while and she'll go over the rest of the clinical trial paperwork with me. Mary? This is the first I've heard of anyone named Mary. Dr. Morganstern seems surprised that I don't know about her. I ask where her office is so I can go there when the EKG is done. He tells me her office is in Burlington, that he just called her and she's driving up here even as we speak. I'm speechless for a minute, especially when I look out the window and see that it's snowing heavily. I don't know who this Mary is but she's driving up Route 128 in a snowstorm to meet with me about the clinical trial. I'm very impressed.

When she arrives, I immediately like her. She finds an office that no one is using and proceeds to tell me that her job is to oversee all of the clinical trial patients. Her dark wavy hair is pulled back with a simple black band; her brown eyes are warm and expressive. She's the type of woman who looks beautiful without make-up. I sit very still and listen to her going on and on about her job, the other patients, the weather today. When it's my turn, I find that she listens as intently as she speaks. I am delighted, and more than a little awed. The Universe has dropped yet another angel in my path.

She tells me about one of Dr. Karp's patients who is knitting him a sweater during the times she waits for her appointments with him. I've never had to wait for him, I tell her, but if I did it would only be because of how he takes the time to sit with his patients and answer all of their questions, not rushing them. I feel good about asserting this because it's a piece of information about me that I'm sharing. I'm trying to say *this is who I am*. This is how I'm dealing with this, trying to shift things around to see the positive. I believe she understands that this is what I'm trying to communicate. And I do feel passionate about being this way. It's one of the things I like best about myself.

Talking with her some more about Dr. Karp, I come to realize that he is the only surgeon on staff who specializes in breast cancer. I am overwhelmed with an extraordinary sense of being blessed, as I remember the day I was told I needed an appointment with a breast surgeon. That was my lucky day, the day they made that appointment for me with Dr. Karp instead of one of the eight general surgeons on staff here. Mary also tells me that until Dr. Karp came to Lahey in October, the hospital never used to participate in clinical trials. The formalized research they're involved in now is because of him.

The strength of the blessing washes over me again, along with the strange thought- *if I had to have breast cancer I guess this was the best year for it.*

When I get back to work, I'm busy finishing several projects so I can turn everything over to John. It definitely feels strange knowing that today is my last day here for several months. I have always hated goodbyes, and today is no exception

Later this afternoon, our Associate Producer and Artistic Director come downstairs to join us. I've always felt a mutual respect and admiration for both of these men. They're usually too busy to stop by the Box Office very often, so when they do we always make time for them. For a moment, I'm thinking they've come to tell us something about this year's Broadway season, but then it becomes clear that they are here to say good-bye to me. Their words of support and kindness touch me deeply, and I stumble through a thank you which is difficult because I'm trying so hard not to cry.

I try to be nonchalant when 5:00 comes and I have to say good-bye to Joan and Jessica and John. They each come to me in their own way and say good-bye. Jessica, a new employee, has some sweet words to say about how she's enjoyed working with me this month and is looking forward to working with me again when I come back. Joan gives me a strong hug and some warm words about taking care and being in touch. John hugs me briefly and says he knows I will get through this just fine. I drive away from the theatre with tears streaming down my face. I feel warm and blessed... and very, very sad.

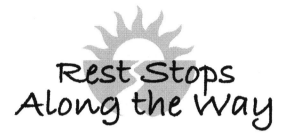

CHAPTER TWELVE

Rest Stops Along the Way

A traveler am I, and a navigator,
and every day I discover a new region within my soul.
— Kahlil Gibran

Tuesday February 12

Standing at the kitchen window in a pool of pale winter sun, I watch the birds flitting to and from the feeder. It feels so good to just *stand* here for several minutes, sipping my decaf. Nothing to do. Nowhere to go.

After a while, I move to the loveseat in the family room where Sasha immediately hops up and settles herself into a black velvet nest on my lap. I savor the goodness of her small weight against my body. My morning is free and I am choosing to sit still with my journal.

I can hardly believe that I don't have to go to work for months and months. It doesn't feel strange to be sitting here in my pajamas and robe instead of getting dressed and driving to work today. It feels perfectly correct, the best gift in the world. But I have to remind myself: it's a gift that comes with strings attached- chemotherapy and radiation treatments. I may be sick some days but in the long run it's going to increase my survival odds, so it's worth it. *I'm* worth it. One book that I read suggested thinking of the chemo as what it's doing *for* me rather than *to* me. I hope I can remember this when the worst is upon me.

Is all of this really happening to me? It's only been two months since Dr. Karp told me there were cancerous cells in my breast tissue. Two months. And my whole world has been turned upside down and shaken since then. I would have thought that this could only be a bad thing, but now I think sometimes our worlds need to be tilted and whirled a bit. I think if I look at it the right way, it can be good for my soul. It does indeed feel like there are angels inside of me, moving the furniture around.

Mary calls this afternoon and tells me I've been "randomized" (who knew this was a *verb?*) into Arm 2 of the clinical trial. Because of this, I'll have four treatments, with all three of the drugs each time. The best thing about this is that I'll be getting the maximum amounts of all of the drugs, including Taxotere (which Dr. Karp once told me he would want *his* wife to have if she ever had breast cancer). Good, I think. That should cover all the bases.

At the video store later, I stand for a long time in the New Releases section, longing to see something that is in any way related to what I'm going through. All I see are romantic comedies (which I usually like) and intense dramas that try my patience just reading the titles.

The only movie I can relate to here is *Wit* featuring Emma Thompson, an actress I admire. I've heard of this film. It's the true story of Vivian Bearing, a college professor who had Stage IV ovarian cancer. I wonder briefly if this is a good idea, renting a movie about a woman dying from cancer. But I gather my courage, hand over the money, and walk to my car clutching the box. When I get home, I set it on the bed, still uncertain if I'm really going to let myself watch it. I do some chores and eye it suspiciously for a few hours, giving it a wide berth, before actually watching it.

My whole being is alive with curiosity and I find I can't turn it off. In some ways, the story is very sad because Vivian has no family or friends to help her through the singular process of dying. No, that's not right. She has family and friends, but she's told them all to stay away. I wonder what I would do in this situation. Would I push everyone away or would I want to have them near me? I hope and pray I'd be brave enough for the latter.

She is quite alone throughout the movie, except for a nurse, and her two doctors (not at all like mine). She's quite alone as she's vomiting, as she's waiting in the dark. She forms a bond with her nurse who is the only medical professional in the movie who truly cares about her.

Near the end of the movie, I see another person who truly cares. It is her former colleague, Dr. Ashford, retired but back in town to see her great grandchild. She offers to recite a John Donne poem and is surprised when Vivian (a former English professor) feebly protests. So Dr. Ashford reaches into her bag, pulls out a children's book, *The Runaway Bunny*, and reads this to her instead.

It's one of those books that preschool children love to hear again and again because of the repetition, and because they instinctively know that the bunny is loved. In the middle of the story, Dr. Ashford lowers the book and looks directly at Vivian. She likens the book to an allegory of the soul, acknowledging that wherever the soul hides, God will find it. Vivian is now so close to death that she can no longer talk, but her eyes speak volumes as she gazes at her friend. Yes, it is clear that she knows this too. There has been no talk of God before this, but there doesn't need to be words when speaking of the soul.

When Dr. Ashford puts down the book, Vivian closes her eyes and quietly breathes her last breath.

By now I'm sobbing into my squished-up pillow. Jeff comes out of his study and a worried look crosses his usually calm features. He asks if I'm ok. He knew I was watching this and I could see from the look on his face when he saw what I'd rented that he thought I just might be out of my mind, but he didn't say anything then and he doesn't say anything now, simply hands me some more tissue. I know he probably thinks I'm crying because I'm watching this woman die, thinking that it could be *me* someday, but that's not it exactly.

The depth of my sadness is coming from the fact that she had to die alone. It wasn't necessary. I know that women die from breast cancer also, and it's certainly crossed my mind (more than once) that it could be *me* someday. But if that ever *is* me, I'm not going to be alone at the end. I have so much love around me now, I know it can get me through anything, even the profound transition that is death.

Wednesday February 13

Lots of people have told me how well they think I'm "dealing" with all of this, how I'm not acting like a victim like some women do when they're told they have breast cancer. Well, I've never felt like a victim, and no one in any time or any way has ever treated me like one. That may have something to do with it.

A while ago I found an Olivia Newton-John song from her album *GAIA*, which consists of songs that she wrote soon after her own breast cancer diagnosis and surgery. The song is called *Why Me*, but basically she is saying "why NOT me?"

And that is exactly how I feel about it. I didn't ask for this and I surely don't want it, but I have it, so I'm going with the flow of it, accepting each moment as it comes, just taking it one step at a time and doing the next thing. Somewhere deep inside me I know that it's not going to get the best of me, that it's only making me stronger, and that it's changing the direction of my life from the inside out. And that can only be a good thing.

Friday February 15

An email from a theatre friend leads me to think more about visualization. I told him I have been visualizing the drugs that will be flowing through my body as clear potent healing energy, and I will continue to do that. But now I feel challenged to do more of it, and more intensely, more consciously. I used visualization to lower my anxiety before my first surgery when I imagined everyone I know who loved me surrounding me in the O.R. that day. And now I'm thinking that I can do the same during my chemo treatments. I like this idea very much.

I email Elizabeth and ask her if she used visualization during her journey. Tonight I receive a reply from her that encourages me to continue what I've started. She says that the most powerful visualization that she uses to this day is the image of herself as an old woman, surrounded by grandchildren, laughing with joy and hugging them with delight. I love this image! And I'm intrigued by the thought of imagining myself an old woman, and what a powerful message that image will send to my spirit and my inner healer.

Saturday February 16

My mind is swirling with mixed thoughts and emotions on the way to the wig salon with JoAnn and Connie. Part of me feels distressed. I can't escape the fact that we're only on this excursion because my hair is going to fall out soon. There's no way I'm looking forward to this. And yet, I feel a curious excitement to be allowed an opportunity to choose a new hairstyle for the next several months. JoAnn and Connie are being extremely kind and supportive; I allow their love to wash over and through me. I allow the excitement to take precedence in my mind.

The owners of the salon, an older married couple, put me at ease right away. The woman has been through cancer so they both know exactly what I'm going through, and their consideration and gentleness shine brightly on me.

They seat me on a high stool in a private room with many large mirrors. The husband comes in, looks at me from several angles, then informs us that he doesn't have any wigs similar to my current hairstyle. He sounds a little worried, which makes me wonder if most women want a wig that looks exactly like their own hair so that no one will notice. I smile and tell him it's perfectly okay because I want something different. He looks again at my wavy brown hair and asks if I'm thinking of curly or straight. I say I'm open to anything.

The next hour is a wild blur of wigs. The owners bring me one after another and we look at my head from all angles, discussing the pros and cons. JoAnn and Connie even try on a few! JoAnn looks especially ravishing in one that is a deep shade of auburn with long sultry waves. I pause, wig in my hand, to absorb this moment. On one hand, this feels like a fun outing with friends. I know why we're here: I have cancer, and I'm going to lose my hair. But somehow, the reason we're here no longer seems as disastrous as it sounds. The reason we're here seems less related to cancer and more connected with friendship, with love. I take a mental snapshot of this moment, store it in my mind for a day when the world feels bleak and lonely.

We all finally agree on a light brown curly style that isn't too long or too short. It seems just right, but the owner doesn't like the color on me. He disappears into the next room, where the wigs are kept, ordered and numbered in long thin white boxes. He returns with a straight wig in his hands and asks me to try it on because he thinks this color will look better on me, but he wants to see it against my skin first.

I take it from his hands and we all admire the color, which the label says is "marbled honey." I put on the wig and toss my head to let it settle. This one is a straight layered cut down to my neck, with long bangs in front. We all stare at my reflection for a moment in the huge mirror. I smile and slowly say what everyone is thinking, that this wig is perfect for me, much better than the other one.

I look at myself in the mirror much longer than necessary. My hair has always been curly, wavy, sometimes frizzy. It's always been difficult to "manage" my hair; I've had my share (and then some) of bad hair days. When I was in my teens and twenties, sometimes I would blow it dry straight, but it never got as straight as this!

We all agree. The cut and color are perfect for my face. I feel better about myself while wearing it, and know instinctively that it will take the sting out of losing my hair if I know I can look this wonderful every day in spite of being bald.

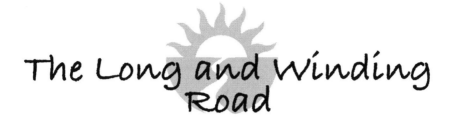

CHAPTER THIRTEEN

The Long and Winding Road

To get through the hardest journey we need take only one step at a time,
but we must keep on stepping.
— Chinese Proverb

Monday February 18

The sky is a cloudless brilliant blue this morning, the day of my first chemo treatment. I hold Jeff's hand tighter than usual as we make our way from the parking lot to the hospital. I shiver a little in the brittle cold, and slowly become aware of a cloud of butterflies in my stomach, remembering the sheer terror I felt before the biopsy (was that only ten weeks ago?). This quivering nervousness is nothing compared to that abrasive fear, only a distant shadowy cousin. But I listen to it nonetheless, curious. What exactly am I afraid of? Only the unknown, what might happen to my body once the drugs take hold. I remember approaching this building for both of my surgeries where I had to relinquish control of my body, my life. And so here I am again today, once again surrendering control. I guess it gets a little easier each time I practice letting go.

I'm not afraid of the treatment itself, for I've been very well prepared by Dr. Morganstern, and by Dawn and Elizabeth and the many women's stories I've read in books and online. I know where I'm going this morning, and I know the people who'll be with me. The security of that has lessened my fear somewhat.

A few weeks ago I bought a special tote bag for my frequent hospital visits, and I'm carrying it today. It's lavender with beautiful images of women's faces in bright fuchsia and turquoise and violet. My heart gladdens every time I look at it. There are other tote bags I could have brought with me but this one is special. This one is a gift to myself, in honor of the courage and heart I'm bringing to this new experience.

While waiting for the blood tests, I pull out the novel I've brought with me. Jeff is sitting quietly beside me, reading *Newsweek*. My bookmark is right there where I left it, a bookmark that I made yesterday at my art table. It's a simple lavender card on which I've handwritten some affirmations. My own affirmations that I have created just for today. I read them now, slowly, breathing deeply before and after each one.

I am filled with healing white light. I picture the liquid drugs flowing into me as white light, dissolving on contact any stray cancer cells that might remain in my body. This clear friendly light courses through my veins, flooding me with distinct radiance.

My immune system is fully functioning, healthy, and strong. I am imagining each bone like a little factory with the factory workers churning out the white blood cells necessary for good immune system action. Some of the factory workers are falling down sick as the chemo works its maddening way through my body, but then they get back up again and go back to "work." And there are countless healthy factory workers, churning out the necessary number of white blood cells.

I am safe. I know that my body, mind and spirit are being protected, monitored, and cared for in ways beyond what I can see and feel in this moment. I believe that I am psychologically, spiritually, and physically safe. My trust and faith are anchored in this belief.

Hands larger than mine are guiding me through this and every journey. I am not alone. I am not doing any of this alone. Divine hands are holding me, stroking my shoulders, cradling my head. Feminine hands, Masculine hands. Hands that have always held me. Hands that know me better than I know myself.

I am well-loved. I am surrounded by people who love and care

for me. I turn the lavender bookmark over now and read the names of every single person who cares for me and is praying for or beaming positive energy to me right now. I bring them with me consciously today for the singular purpose of alleviating my anxiety and assisting with the healing. I smile as I name them silently, realizing it's getting very crowded in this small waiting room!

Soon the preliminary blood work and physical exam are finished and I am in the "sunroom" in the back of the oncology center. Dr. Morganstern has given it this euphemistic label because the entire length of the back wall is floor-to-ceiling windows facing west. Right now the space is flooded with light, and I like how this gives the area a broader, cheerier look. One might never guess that cancer warfare happens here on a regular basis.

I've been seated in a large gray reclining chair with a soft pillow at my back. There's a small metal table on wheels nearby and I place my new tote bag on it so it's within reaching distance. If I close my eyes, I can just barely pretend that I'm in an airplane getting ready for take-off. Let's see…. Where shall we go today?

But my nurse (Ellie) has other ideas. She matter-of-factly hands me several papers and brochures, and begins to go through the information with me. It feels like she's trying to prepare me for a test I've already studied enough for, but I try to pay attention anyway. Ellie is a little older than me, with pretty blonde hair and a kind face. I like her straightforwardness and I like her smile which offers empathy rather than pity. She talks her way through the information for an hour and I nod continually while she speaks. We cover all the bases: nausea, nutrition, hair loss and fatigue.

By the time she's finished, it's 11:00 and she gives me an anti-nausea pill in a cup. I kiss Jeff good-bye and reassure him I'll be fine as he leaves to do the grocery shopping. Then Ellie preps my hand for the IV. I'm surprised. I thought it was going into the crook of my arm, where the blood tests are done. She's extremely careful with the needle, especially when she sees the black and blue shadows that are still on the back of my hand from the IV mishap during my first surgery. She talks nonstop the entire time she is preparing me, and in another lifetime I might have found this carefree chatter annoying, to say the least. But today, in this new life I seem to have acquired, I find myself infinitely fascinated with stories of her family, the weather, and the latest movies she's seen.

The first drug I receive is the bright red adriamycin which glistens like cherry Kool-aid in the plastic bag that hangs from the top of the IV stand. Ellie stays with me the entire 15 minutes, administering it by hand, ever so slowly squeezing the syringe into my vein. She tells me she's doing it this way to be sure none of it seeps out through the IV and onto my skin. I try not to think about what this means- if it's too dangerous to touch my skin, what is it doing to the inside of me?

Next she hooks me up to a bag of the crystal clear cytoxan, then rushes away, leaving me to my book for a total of five minutes. When she pops back in the room to check on me, she's talking about lunch.

Lunch? I can actually *eat* while I'm having chemo? Why didn't anyone tell me this? I check in with myself and realize that I'm actually hungry, so I say yes to the tuna sandwich on wheat bread and the split pea soup. I eat half of the sandwich which tastes surprisingly good.

When the cytoxan bag is empty, a shrill beeper sounds insistently, and Ellie comes right back to me. I ask her to unhook me from the IV so I can go to the bathroom down the hall. When I return, it's time for the taxotere, also a clear liquid suspended in a bag on the IV pole. She tells me that the taxotere will take about an hour, but she comes back every fifteen minutes to take my temperature, pulse, and blood pressure. It seems that this is the most potent of the three drugs, requiring extra caution to be sure my body is absorbing it without any repercussions.

Jeff comes back during this final round and I give him the pea soup and crackers while I eat the rest of the sandwich. It's comforting to have him beside me again. We talk about everything but the fact that I'm sitting in a hospital with drugs coursing through my body because I have cancer.

By 1:15 it's over and I'm giddy with relief. I can't believe how normal I feel. It's almost as if nothing's happened at all. I know they told me most people don't throw up during chemo, but I never quite believed them.

At home, I help Jeff put away the groceries. I'm still feeling really good, so I make a huge pot of spinach lentil soup, our favorite. We had it a year ago while eating out, and then I searched and sleuthed until I found the recipe online. It is unbelievably delicious. I'm thinking this will be a great, healthy meal for these upcoming days when my body is trying to recover from the chemo assault. I take a mugful upstairs so I can eat while emailing Dawn and Elizabeth the good news that I've survived the first treatment.

After an hour of sitting at the computer, I begin to feel a little ragged around the edges. Fatigue looms on the horizon. I quickly grab my coat and head to the grocery store around the corner for a few things that Jeff forgot earlier. And flowers. I'm definitely feeling the need for flowers right now.

I'm moving much more slowly when I get back. "Good" and "normal" are no longer words I know the meaning of. I put the groceries away, plunk the dark purple tulips in a tall crystal vase which I carry upstairs (was it always this heavy?). I dare these flowers to make me think of spring, or anything besides the miserable way I'm feeling right now. I throw my clothes in a heap by the bed, toss on a warm nightgown, and crawl under the covers.

No, this is definitely not normal. It's 5:30 on a Monday afternoon and I'm lying in bed with my nightgown on, huddled under the comforter begging for sleep. I take an anti-nausea pill even though I'm not exactly feeling nauseous. Ellie has told me to do this and I am more than happy to do as she says. As the night progresses, I feel like there is nausea just beneath the surface of my awareness. Perhaps the pills are deadening my body's inclination to vomit. I feel blah and icky, like a limp dishrag just waiting to be wrung out. It feels good to just lie here and let Jeff wait on me, which he gladly does. He makes me an omelet and toast, brings me water and a Popsicle, lays beside me and wraps his arms around me for comfort and support. I tell him he missed his calling and should go into nursing. He laughs and rubs my back. I wonder how I would get through this without him.

He has to leave for a few hours to help a client with their taxes. When he gets back, I move to the other side of the bed so I can lay on my right side and wrap my arms around him. I know this pleases him because we haven't lain like this in a long time. A very long time. I feel like I'm absorbing some of his strength and energy into my very flesh and bones. Spooning like this feels excruciatingly good, and brings me to tears. I let them flow and Jeff continues to hold me, rocking me, stroking my back, murmuring words of love and support, reminding me that everything is going to be all right.

Wednesday February 20

I don't have the energy for much today except reading. I feel confined to my bed and yet it feels like a luxury to be able to sit still for hours at a time and read as much as I want. I'm deeply tired and there is a strange metallic taste in my mouth. I don't feel hungry, but I find myself chewing on different kinds of food simply to see if the metallic taste will go away. It doesn't. Even water tastes bad; I simply can't drink it. This worries me because I know I'm supposed to be drinking lots of water. But then I remember Ellie telling me that Popsicles, soda, juice, and even ice cream count as liquids so I try a bottle of root beer and an orange Popsicle instead. The sweetness is a gift.

My sense of smell has also heightened considerably. Last night I made honey mustard chicken, but could only eat a few bites because the scent of mustard seemed overpowering to me. I had to go downstairs after dinner and spray room deodorizer in the kitchen because the smell was making me nauseous.

I religiously take the anti-nausea pills every six hours, and they must be working because I haven't thrown up once. I don't exactly feel nauseous, just really icky. My energy is at a very low ebb, and I can fall asleep much quicker than I ever have before.

I'm reading *Every Good and Perfect Gift*, a novel by Brenda Jernigan. Reading some more of it this afternoon, my heart is caught by something the main character says about living in the midst of their calling. This, *this* is exactly what I want! To be alive, and in the center of my calling. Like the way Mary, the research assistant, is so totally full of joy to be doing what she's doing, and how that joy spills over to her patients. The way my friend Christina used to blaze with happiness when she talked of her life, her marriage, her teaching. I've had this aliveness before. I've had the glow that comes from being in the right place, doing exactly what I'm meant to do. I had it when I first started teaching, when I started the educational consulting work, when I was creating and leading the teacher workshops, when I was at St. Peter's in Salem, when I first got together with Jeff and his children, and when I first started at the theatre.

But right now on my journey, I'm not living in the midst of any calling, or at least that's how it feels. I've been going to my job at the theatre every day and that's all it's felt like for the last year or so- a job. It feels empty, vacuous to look at it this way. I wonder if I'll want to go back when these treatments are over. Being away from the theatre for a change, being on the outside looking in, is giving me a new perspective. Right now I can honestly say I don't miss it at all. Oh, I miss the people, the camaraderie we have, the friendships, the feeling of having a second home. But I don't miss the stress, the aggravation, the negativity that sometimes flourishes there.

I know I don't need to decide anything immediately and I'm grateful for this. I'm willing to be patient, to let time teach me what it will about this job, about my life. Perhaps my calling right now is to gather my inner strength and fight the cancer. Or maybe my calling is to step back for a few months and listen, simply listen to my inner yearnings and then give myself permission to follow them.

Thursday February 21

This morning I sleep until 10:00 and take a bath instead of a shower. This is the most strenuous thing I've done so far all week. It's a foreign feeling, being so continually and easily depleted of energy in spite of hours of unbroken rest. The threat of nausea is beginning to lessen its ironclad grip on me. I feel much less queasy today.

One thing I desperately need to do today is get rid of that spinach soup I made on Monday. I'm certain I will never make it again. Just looking at the six plastic tubs of it in the refrigerator makes me want to vomit and I'm slightly amused because I *love* that soup. Used to love that soup. I can't even stand the thought of opening the containers and dumping the soup out in the sink, watching all those slimy green lentils sliding down the drain. So I carry the plastic cartons out to the back deck and happily dump them in the trash. A week ago I would have been worried about throwing out all that plastic instead of recycling. Today, I simply don't care.

Later I am reading *Every Good and Perfect Gift* again, and one of the characters is talking about pilgrimages being a matter of sore feet. My heart again is jostled awake by this author's words. Pilgrimages and journeys are about serious footwork, not just about the love and joy that you find along the way. That's all well and good, sure. But you won't be finding the joy if you're not putting one foot in front of the other, step after step after tedious step.

And that is what I'm doing on this journey, I realize. Simply doing the next thing, taking the next step. Resting in that, and then taking *another* step, doing the *next* thing. My "feet" do indeed feel sore, but this doesn't mean I'm not walking hand in hand with Spirit.

CHAPTER FOURTEEN

Embracing the Desert

I haven't a clue as to how my story will end. But that's all right.
When you set out on a journey and night covers the road,
you don't conclude that the road has vanished.
And how else could we discover the stars?
— Unknown

Friday February 22

Today is the first day I've felt fairly "normal," although I'm probably losing any sense of what that actually means. Last night I was able to stay awake until midnight to watch the women's Olympic skating competition, and in spite of that I woke up at 7:30 this morning, ready to start the day. All week I've been sleeping ten to twelve hours at night with additional naps in the afternoon (just like our cats!). It felt so wonderful to be able to stay up late last night and still get up early this morning.

I'm only just beginning to get used to the fact that I have abundant time on my hands now. Time. Real, true time. I've had almost two weeks of it already and can hardly believe that I still have many more yet to come. Seventeen weeks. Eighty-five days. Time for me and me alone. When was the last time I had this?

I've been asking myself another question a lot lately- what *is* truly next for me? Can I really go back to the theatre? Do I even *want* to go back there? Right now I honestly don't know what is next, but I'm promising myself that I will try and relax *into* the answer, and not struggle so much to see ahead. And I've turned my question into an affirmation of trust: *I am finding my way to what is next.*

I had a dream last week, and in the dream I'm near the end of my radiation treatments. It's almost time to go back to work. I'm waiting for Robert our Stage Manager to come back from vacation so I can ask him if he'll let me work backstage in June. In the dream, it's a burning desire, a passionate question. I'm wanting to do what my niece Stephanie did last summer during her internship at the theatre: helped with costumes, ran props around during the show, assisted the stage management team with scenery changes.

The dream confuses me; I can't quite grasp what it means. Do I really want to work *backstage* at the theatre? I don't think that's it exactly. Perhaps the dream represents my desire to be more connected to the creative side of my life, since the production side of theatre work is more associated with creativity than the box office. If someone were to ask me what I want (right now, this moment), I'd say not to go back to "work" at all, anywhere. To simply to be able to stay home and write, create my note cards and maybe even figure out a way to sell them.

But is this just the chemo talking, or is this really me?

If I could have exactly what I wanted, it would be this utter stillness I feel right now, day after day, morning after morning. Sitting at my desk, writing my heart out onto empty pages, the window open, birds and seagulls calling in the distance, the slow pace of an easy morning.

But reality intervenes; I must drive myself to Lahey for my daily neupogen shot. Ellie chats with me cheerfully while she swabs my thigh with alcohol, then gently jabs the needle in. I have to have this shot every day because it keeps my white blood cell count up, helping to counteract the side effects of the taxotere. If everything goes well, I'll soon be able to give myself the shots at home.

Saturday February 23

Today I wake up with no metallic taste in my mouth and a good amount of energy, all of which fills me with clean happiness. Perhaps I'm going to fly through this chemo thing without as many side effects as we anticipated. I actually feel normal again.

I go to Lahey for my daily shot, then to a nearby flower shop for some perfect buttery yellow daffodils. How they make me smile.

My next stop is A.C. Moore, one of my favorite places in the world. Ordinarily I can spend hours wandering the aisles, fingering the ribbon and yarn, admiring the papers and rubber stamps, letting my imagination fly from one project to another, trying to decide what to buy with my 40% off coupon. But today I find myself moving slower and slower, feeling suddenly weak and very tired. I feel sad as I slip the coupon back into my pocket and drive home. A.C. Moore will have to wait.

Jeff and I were going to go to the movies later and then to our favorite Mexican restaurant, but I can tell this isn't going to happen. It seems I've already used up my energy allotment for the day. I feel so discouraged. The only thing giving me a bit of hope is the vase of daffodils on my dark wood dresser. They smile at me gently, reminding me of brighter days. They remind me that I'm not an invalid even though I'm lying in bed day after day in homage to this illness that has caught me unaware.

So much for feeling normal.

Sunday February 24

My stomach is feeling quaky and strange even though it's been twelve days since my treatment. Maybe it's because I've been eating more dairy than usual, or maybe it's the antibiotic I have to take because of the neupogen shots. Whatever. I refuse to worry about it any longer. There are worse things I could be experiencing.

My head is starting to itch, which means my hair is going to start falling out very soon. I am thinking this thought, and I know it's real, but it still seems foreign to me, like it's happening to someone else.

I'm thinking of trying to find a therapist, a woman therapist, maybe even one who's had breast cancer. A woman who can help me through this. Mostly what I need help with is my relationship with Jeff. Whenever he reaches out to me, especially in bed, I can't seem to stop crying. It just feels so good to have him there beside me, but then I start feeling a mother lode of guilt because my need for sexual contact has completely flown the coop. I've read that some women feel contaminated from the chemo, but that's not it. It's more like I feel physically handicapped, not to mention the fact that between the surgery and the constant fatigue, I just don't feel like myself anymore.

We talked about all of this last night and he kept reassuring me that we don't need to make love to feel close, that he loves me as I am, and that this will all be over soon. I'm so afraid that he's going to leave me. That he's going to get tired of this, tired of me, and look for "entertainment" elsewhere. I'm sure Jeff isn't like that but I'm still aware of a few tiny doubts lurking catlike in the back of my mind, ready to pounce on my slightest negative thought. But I wonder….. is it Jeff that I'm doubting, or is it me?

Monday February 25

As tired as I feel, I don't want to miss the first support group meeting at Lahey. Pam, the social worker, explained that it's more of a psycho-educational group, that there will be information given and shared. We won't just be sitting around sharing our woes. This in itself has been enough to get me to the meeting. When I've thought of breast cancer support groups, I've imagined bald women who look weak and scared and pale, women who are crying, women whose stories are too difficult to listen to. I don't think a gathering like that would be helpful for me.

There's one woman already in the meeting room when I arrive, plus the intern who's working with Pam this semester. I notice that the intern only listens unless we specifically draw her into the conversation. I wonder if she's shy, or if she was instructed to let us do all the talking. Two other women join us. We sit around a large rectangular table and tell our stories, one by one.

It feels incredibly good to be in a room with other women who've been through what I've just been through. Their stories are similar with shades of detail that make each one unique. Bonita is already halfway through her chemo treatments. She's wearing a purple scarf tonight but is telling stories about her wig that make us laugh. At one point she says that the hardest time for her was when her hair was falling out, because she had to look in the mirror and *face the fact of her illness*. I am startled by this confession, want to stop the flow of her story, argue with her. This isn't how I see it at all. I feel like the cancer in me was completely removed during that second surgery, that it's not inside me anymore. I think the chemo I'm getting now is just insurance that there won't be any more cancer, and that losing my hair is the price I have to pay for that insurance.

But I don't interrupt her, for she is telling her story and I want to honor every woman's experience, whether I agree with what she says or not. I'm happy to tell my story as well. Although I've shared online several times, this is the first time I've spoken it out loud and it feels immeasurably good. The others offer me affirmative nods and smiles while I speak. I feel seen and heard, but I keep wishing that Dawn and Elizabeth were here. I've forgotten how long it takes to bond with people emotionally in "real time" as opposed to cyberspace, where I bonded with Dawn and Elizabeth so quickly due to the speed and immediate intimacy of email.

Wednesday February 27

Dr. Morganstern tells me that my white blood cell count is "sky high." This means I don't need to come in for the next three neupogen shots. I feel excited and happy about this. Happy and free! I can collage or read or write all morning if I want to tomorrow, and not be disrupted with the trip to the hospital for the shot.

I feel so good today. I don't dare use the word "normal" anymore, but I do feel good. No stomach cramps, no soft bowel movements, no lethargy. I'm thinking of going to a movie this afternoon but it's very cold and windy out, so maybe I'll just stay in and finish a few card projects. Dawn's doctor has told her to stay away from crowded places because of increased risk of catching a cold or other virus. I ask Dr. Morganstern about this and he kindly says not to worry about it.

After washing his hands in the sink, he casually asks how my spirit is these days. This startles me, makes me sit up straighter. No doctor in my forty-six year history has ever been remotely interested in my spirit (or if they were, they didn't ask). We've just spent fifteen minutes reviewing my symptoms. He's asked me every conceivable question about how my body reacted last week and how it's feeling today. And now he's asking me if my *spirit* is well also.

I am in awe that he has asked me this, and reply that my spirit is doing well. If I'd come in here today feeling poorly in any way, I'd have broken down and cried right here in this chilly little room in my dorky hospital gown. The simple fact of the question itself has touched me and lifted my spirits. Here is another example of a good hospital being a true blend of technology and tenderness. If I wasn't sure about my relationship with Dr. Morganstern before today, I am now. He is my oncologist and I would not trade him for all the craft supplies in the world.

Thursday February 28

A bright and windy day shines through the window as I settle myself at the kitchen table, warm in my sweatpants and large red sweater. A bagel with jelly, a mug of decaf with cream, and my empty journal laden with possibilities are spread out before me, along with several half-finished art projects. What shall I do today? The thought of all this uncluttered *time* ahead of me is very healing.

I could do this writing, this dreaming, in my Quiet Room but it's located in the smallest room in our house, and crammed in there are my writing desk and files, an art table and all my art supplies, my favorite blue rocking chair by the window, and a small altar. I feel crowded now when I go in there, and I'm longing for a bigger space to spread out a bit.

There's a larger room down the hall that technically belongs to Amanda and Merri. But Amanda is living with her boyfriend, Merri is living with Jeff's sister, and day after day that room sits empty. I go in there this morning after breakfast and savor the sunshine flooding in through the east window. If we could just move all of Amanda's stuff (and Merri's bunk beds) out of here and down into the largest empty room on the lower level, I could move my Quiet Room in here. Amanda and Merri could share the bigger room downstairs whenever they come to visit.

This thought fills my soul with immediate joy, in spite of the thought of the hours it will take us to move this stuff out and my stuff in. I can imagine the room empty, completely empty. I can picture it painted in deep shades of teal and aqua. My desk will go over there in the corner and I'll put the altar right here in front of the window. I'll have two long art tables on the opposite side, and there will be just enough room for a comfy chair against the remaining wall.

I will talk about this tonight with Jeff and see if he will help me turn these possibilities into reality.

Friday March 1

Just the thought of moving my Quiet Room into the new space fills me with excitement, a feeling that I stop and savor because I haven't felt it once these past few months. I *have* felt: fear, gratitude, anxiety, grief, anger and joy…. but not this bubbling-from-the-depths-of-me *excitement*. It's taking some of the sting out of how strange my body feels these days, some of the dread out of my imminent hair loss. I am acutely aware of the fact that having things to look forward to is one of the best medicines I can give myself right now.

Amanda calls to say she's coming to get the rest of her things tomorrow. Now all we need to do is dismantle the bunk beds and move them downstairs. Jeff agrees to do this. Merri is here for the weekend and I ask her tonight if she'd mind having the downstairs room when she moves in with us this summer. We talk about how it's bigger and how she'll have more privacy. She says she likes that room and doesn't mind at all. I'm hoping she really means it and isn't just saying it because she thinks it's what I want to hear. What I really hope is that she doesn't care which room is hers, as long as she has one, as long as we want her to live with us, and God knows (and I hope she does too) we do.

Saturday March 2

I'm feeling very down today, in a major funk. However, I feel considerably better than last night when I was heading straight into depression. I guess there are levels to this misery, levels that I never knew existed because I never felt like this so long before. I don't know how to share any of this with Jeff because some of it has to do with him, with us. How we don't *talk* anymore, how we just sit and watch TV at night until he falls asleep in the recliner and leaves me sitting alone in the bed, propped up against an acre of pillows. I HATE THIS. I spend all day alone and then he comes home after work and I *still* feel like I'm spending time alone.

I've been wondering if maybe I should have kept working a little bit, just a few hours a week. So much of my social life is based at the theatre. I'm feeling cut off now, like I'm not a part of it anymore. I know I can go back to visit, but I'm afraid they'll be thinking I could've kept on working if I can drop in from time to time. It's so silly, I know. Why do I always worry so much about what others think?

For instance, yesterday afternoon when I saw Maggie in the grocery store, I avoided her. This is bothering me today. I have loved Maggie ever since she came to work at the theatre two years ago. She's the sweetest woman in the world. So why did I turn my cart in the other direction and leave the store immediately as soon as I saw her in my aisle? I'm not exactly ashamed of having breast cancer, but I *am* quite sick of talking about it all the time. No, that's not it exactly. What I'm tired of is worrying about how much the other person already knows, and how much I should tell them, and how they're going to take the news, and how I need to reassure them that I'm going to be all right. I find this exhausting.

"So? You avoided her," the reasonable, motherly part of me is saying. "So what?"

For once, I listen to this voice within me, and attempt agreement. So what, indeed! I decide right now to stop beating myself up over this incident.

Instead, I start worrying how I'm going to react when my hair starts falling out. Women in the online survivor groups have been telling me how traumatic it was for them. I ask Elizabeth if she cried when she looked at herself in the mirror and saw herself bald the first time, and she says yes. I'm afraid of that, I guess. Becoming ugly, seeing myself as ugly, feeling embarrassed when I ask Jeff to shave my head. I know it's going to happen any day now and I'm extremely anxious about it.

But now that I think about it, who's to say that it has to be that way for me? Maybe I could look at it as one more hurdle to get over before this adventure is through. Maybe I could look at it as a lesson in discovering who I am apart from my appearance. A lesson in remembering, accentuating, and actually *believing in* my inner beauty.

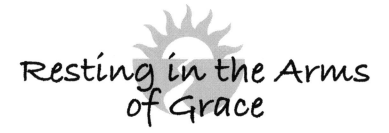

CHAPTER FIFTEEN

Resting in the Arms of Grace

The winds of grace blow all the time.
All we have to do is set our sails.

— Ramakrishna

Wednesday March 6

I'm losing my hair. But it isn't happening the way I thought it would. It's not exactly *falling out*, but appears to be loosening its hold on my head, like it doesn't need me anymore. And I'm at the stage now where it only comes out if I run my fingers through it. Taking a shower is becoming a tedious, time-consuming procedure; strands and strands of my hair keep getting tangled in my fingers and I'm using gallons of water rinsing them all off.

I started wearing the wig yesterday and so far I'm okay with it, although it startles me a little when I catch a glimpse of myself in the mirror.

Who is that stranger with the pale face and honey blonde straight hair? I'm slowly coming to accept that she is me, and I like her, even so.

This morning I drive to the mall and buy two hats for the days when I won't want to wear the wig. They're called "crusher" hats, soft and velvety in my hands. One is dark purple and the other is a leopard print. I like them both. I like how I look in them. I like how they make me feel. Changing my appearance like this (the wig, the hats) has certainly softened the reality of my imminent baldness.

Later this afternoon, anticipating next week's chemo treatment, I call my friend Joan and ask her if she will make a few meals for us next week. That was the hardest thing for me the first time- trying to find the energy to plan and prepare dinner every night. I know Jeff would be satisfied with frozen dinners or canned soup, but I want to give him more than that, and I know I need to be eating better than that too. Joan has been asking me for weeks what she can do to help. Today when I ask her, she is more than happy to comply, and says she'll ask our friend Sheila who works at the theatre too. I call Jeff's mother Connie and ask her to make a few meals as well. I feel a delighted relief when I hang up the phone. One less thing to worry about now.

As I lay in bed on my back tonight, my left arm is propped up on a soft pillow. Will I ever sleep in a normal position again? I listen to the sound of Jeff snoring beside me. Usually I find this irritating but tonight it has a peaceful rhythm to it. Our room is very dark and quiet except for the snoring. Sasha is curled up against my left thigh, sleeping deeply. Once in a while I hear her softly sigh as she shifts her weight against me.

I breathe in the stillness and find myself centered in a way that I have deeply missed for a long time. Once again I sense the presence of Spirit, the essence of Joy, right here filling the room. I cannot see or touch it but it is indeed very real and present. I feel totally calm, completely reassured that I will be able to get through all of these cancer treatments, and that I will emerge from this journey stronger and more sure of who I am.

I breathe slowly as I whisper aloud the names of the people I'm praying for, turning them over to this Spirit, this essence of compassion that has taken up residence here. And I do not forget to name myself. I feel like a little girl, and a warm, nurturing mother is tucking me in, singing me an inner lullaby of love and peace, rocking me into a gentle quiet sleep.

Thursday March 7

I'm having lunch at Bertucci's with my actor friend George. It's so good to see him again, and the hug he gives me is warm and loving. He compliments me greatly on the wig, telling me how wonderful I look, although I know I'm pale and that there are dark shadows under my eyes.

He's driven an hour from New Hampshire, and I've invited Jeff's mom Connie and my friend Joan to join us because they also know George from the theatre. Joan is late joining us. I see her in the entryway, looking for us, and I wave frantically, trying to get her attention. She looks right at me but doesn't recognize me. At first I'm baffled, then I remember the wig, so I go up to her and tap her on the shoulder. She is startled, but then grabs me to her in a hug so ferocious I'm afraid the wig is going to fly right off my head.

As we savor the salad and pasta, I notice that George continually focuses the attention back on me, asking me a multitude of questions. The discussion meanders into the topics of theatre business, vacation plans, and mutual friends, but every time we wander a bit too far down one of these roads, George looks me in the eye and asks another question.

I notice how uncomfortable this feels, probably because I'm not used to such thorough attention, particularly in respect to my cancer. Most people ask me how the treatment went, or how I'm feeling, and are easily appeased with one-word answers. I'm not sure if that's because they don't really want to know much more than that, or if they honestly don't know how to ask.

On the other hand, here is George, asking very specific questions. *How often do you have to have the chemo? Did you feel nauseous after they gave it to you? So, has any of your hair fallen out yet?* I'm slightly amused at his candor. If I give him a one or two word answer, he simply asks more questions to draw the deeper truth from me.

He doesn't bombard me with these questions all at once, but intersperses them throughout the hour we're together. As I answer these intermittent questions, I also am aware that I am feeling quite well-loved and cared-for. In spite of my initial discomfort, I now find his questions endearing. He's only asking because he hasn't seen me in three months and is genuinely interested in what's going on with me.

Tonight as I wait for sleep, I watch my breathing, once again aware of the very near presence of Spirit. It is difficult to name. Perhaps it is Jesus…perhaps an angel. I can't see it with my eyes, but I can certainly feel it in the deepest core of my being. Someone or Something, some loving whole Presence is beside me, waiting to hear about my day. My heart overflows with gratitude and I express thanks for what I noticed today- the purple crocuses beaming in the sunshine outside the library steps, the sound of the gulls when I drove by Dane Street Beach, the short walk I managed to take, Sasha's unconditional, undeniable love, the amusing way Scooter rolls on the brick walk like a dog, the time alone with Jeff tonight, the undeniable fact that I have so many people in my life who love me so much (almost bald or not).

I begin to ask for blessings for the people who grace my life but I feel an inner prompting. *No, my dear,* you *first this time.* So I pause for a moment. What do I want? What do I need? What am I most anxious about tonight, right now, this very moment?

I ask that the sore, ragged cuticle on my left hand not become infected. I ask for the grace and patience to get through all of this. I ask for a lessening of anxiety concerning my hair loss, a way to maybe get used to it a little bit at a time. I also ask that I be allowed to live at least another twenty years. I wonder if this is too presumptuous, then decide that it's not at all too much to ask for.

For one fleeting moment of frozen fear, I wonder if this "Presence" is simply preparation for my imminent death. I can see very easily how comforting it would be to be dying, and to have this Presence beside me, talking me through it, leading me forward through the transition, forward and on to the bigger Journey. I allow the fear to make itself known. I feel it fully in my racing heartbeat, in my dry lips, my jittery stomach. I feel it. I feel it and then I let it go, relaxing into the warmth of this moment, now. For in this moment now I am certainly not dying, and that is all that matters.

Saturday March 9

Jeff and I are at a funky little Bed & Breakfast in Ogunquit, Maine. We're taking this weekend to enjoy some alone time together. We got here yesterday afternoon and have been spending most of our time sleeping and cuddling close in the double bed, reading, and watching TV.

I'm wearing my wig now because I really need to. Last night Jeff used hair clippers to give me a buzz cut. I don't like how it looks, but it's better than pulling out hundreds of strands of hair at a time every morning in the shower.

This afternoon we walk towards the Marginal Way, one of my favorite places in the world. But the wind is powerful, the salt air still bears the penetrating chill of winter, and I'm not as strong as I was the last time we were here. I've tied a long bright scarf over the wig to keep it attached to my head, apprehensive that it will blow off and everyone will see my baldness. Why do I care? I have cancer, for crying out loud. Why does it matter what my head looks like? We only get halfway to the beach when I reluctantly stop. I hate to admit it, but I simply can't go any farther. Jeff puts his arm around me and we head back to the house.

Tonight we order pizza and eat it on the bed as we watch *Everybody Loves Raymond* reruns. The wig observes us from the bedpost; I'm wearing one of the soft cotton head scarves that Dawn sent me. I look almost like myself in it, and it feels like a soft embrace on my scalp. This is sheer delight: giggling with my husband, sharing pizza on a large four-poster bed. I treasure this evening of laughter and love, storing it away in my heart for what I feel certain will be darker times ahead.

Sunday March 10

Jeff's sister Jan has invited us over for dinner. She and her husband Donald greet me with warm hugs and ask me how I'm feeling; they admire the wig. As we dig into the feast Jan has prepared, Donald asks if I'm ready for some more "chemical enhancement" tomorrow (my next chemo treatment) and I laugh so hard that I almost choke on the fruit salad. Wonderfully euphemistic, I'm thinking! And the more laughter the better. This will be something funny to share with Ellie tomorrow, and I notice that this makes me feel happy all over.

Tuesday March 12

I look at myself in the mirror this morning. The buzzed hair is falling out now too. More and more hair, short as it is, goes down the shower drain every day. I sigh and decide to take a bath instead, soaking in vanilla scented oil while reading the latest issue of *Oprah*. Whenever I read this magazine, it seems I'm able to reclaim another missing part of myself.

When I finally make my way downstairs, I find a huge pot of wonderfully fragrant beef stew on the porch, with a note from Joan. I smile at this gift, put it in the fridge, and make myself an English muffin with grape jelly, savoring the sweetness and crunch. Then I slowly climb the stairs and stand beside the bed for a moment, deciding what to do next. My body opts for rest, so I climb back in and pull the covers up and around me. I read all morning, take a three hour nap after lunch, and watch TV all afternoon.

Before Jeff comes home I remove the lavender head scarf and put on the wig and a little bit of make-up. I'm listening to my affirmations tape as I do this, and one of them has caught my attention today. *I am beautiful,* I hear my voice saying on the tape.

I am *beautiful.*

I am beautiful.

I repeat the words aloud because I know I must. I look in the mirror and think maybe I do look a little bit beautiful with the wig on. No, that is not what I meant when I recorded that affirmation. My intention was to remind myself that I'm beautiful no matter what is happening to me on the outside. However, that's pretty difficult to do when my hair is falling out in patches all over the place. Last week I looked pretty good with the buzzcut Jeff gave me. Today I'm not so thrilled when I look in the mirror. My hair is gone.

Jeff doesn't seem to mind at all that I'm pretty much bald. It bothers *me* way more than it bothers him. But then of course, it's my hair, not his. Besides, most of my energy these days is going into napping. There's really not a lot left over for thinking about my hair. They told me it was going to fall out, and so it has. The chemo drugs must be doing their job, killing any cancer cells that might be in my body, as well as my hair follicle cells. Today it seems as simple as that.

Wednesday March 13

This morning it takes every ounce of energy that is left in me (and it doesn't feel like much) to shower, get dressed and drive to Lahey for my appointment with Ellie. She is going to watch me give myself my first Neupo-gen shot. If all goes well, I'll be able to give myself the shots at home from now on.

I walk more slowly than usual, conserving what little strength I have as I make my way from the outer reaches of the parking lot into the hospital. The wind is in high gear again and I hold onto my wig with both hands. As soon as I get inside, I head straight for the bathroom mirror to make sure the wig is hanging straight on my head. When I had my own hair and it got whipped around in the wind on a day like this, I could simply run my fingers through it, fluff it in just the right places and I wouldn't even need a mirror to know that it looked right. I miss those days.

The waiting area is crowded today. Some people are only here for blood tests, I know, but many of them are waiting for their time in the "sun-room" or waiting for loved ones to finish a treatment there. I look around at each of them, sending them silent blessings from my heart. I pull out my paperback novel and attempt to focus on the words.

In a few minutes, I notice Dr. Morganstern walking through the wait-ing area. He heads toward a woman sitting in the back row of chairs. She is tall and thin with ink black straight hair hanging in an angled cut to her chin. Tears are welling up in her beautiful almond eyes as he sits down beside her and asks her how she's doing. I've never met this woman, but I know exactly what she's thinking. She's thinking that he genuinely wants to know *how she is*, that he is not simply making small talk.

Their conversation is quiet but the area is small enough that I can hear some of what they are saying. Her husband has recently died. Dr. Morganstern speaks quietly, gently, and she listens attentively while wiping away her tears. After a few minutes he stands, tenderly touches her shoulder, says "I wish you much strength," and walks back towards his office. Tears burn in my own eyes. He used the same tone of voice when he asked me how my spirit was a few weeks ago. I'm moved once again by his sincerity and compassion.

I am also slightly unnerved. People do *die* from cancer. I stare this fact in the face for a moment, then tuck it away into another corner of my brain. I'm *not* going to let this take control, *not* going to allow it to get the best of me.

And then another aspect of this whole scene startles me as I watch my doctor's white-coated figure disappear behind his office door. People die from cancer, more than I want to know about. I can dismiss this fact and focus on other things, even though I'm fighting this cancer on a daily basis. But what about Dr. Morganstern? How can he dismiss it so easily? How can he dismiss it at all? He must lose patients to cancer occasionally, in spite of how good a doctor he is. How does he stand the pain of that? My admiration for him intensifies and I send a silent blessing his way.

Ellie calls me into the office and I nervously give myself the neupogen shot with her expert coaching. It's fairly simple, really. Swab my upper leg with alcohol, pull up the pre-filled syringe, thrust it firmly into my skin at a ninety degree angle, (there's no blood and I'm amazed at this), release the syringe, put on a small bandage. I'm proud of myself.

At home, I pull off my jeans and sweatshirt, get into my softest blue cotton nightgown and climb gratefully into bed. This little excursion has left me exhausted in body, mind, and spirit. I close my eyes, giving myself over to the necessity of rest.

Thursday March 14

Several half-finished note card designs lay helter-skelter on the table in my Quiet Room, waiting to be mounted onto colored cardstock. I'm anxious to get to work on this, excited at the prospect of getting some finished cards together. But today, all I can do is look at them on the table. I'm just too tired to do too much of anything.

The doorbell rings and it's Sheila from the theatre delivering a casserole. It's good to see her even though I now feel like I'm living on another planet altogether. She tells me that I look wonderful and I thank her, but I can't make myself believe it. I've put on weight, there are dark circles under my eyes, and I'm not wearing make-up. Maybe she expected me to look much worse than this.

I put the dinner casserole in the fridge and begin rummaging for something to eat. Even though it's noon, I'm not hungry yet, but the metallic taste in my mouth is overpowering, much worse than last time. I've begun drinking root beer and ginger ale instead of water. Prior to chemo, I would be condemning myself for drinking high calorie beverages and eating whatever tastes good to me in the moment. But right now, my brain simply can't process the ill effects of so many high calorie/high fat foods. They (and they alone) are able to make this strange taste in my mouth disappear for a few minutes. Prior to chemo, I would never in a million years eat an entire frozen pizza and a bowl of potato chips for lunch, then follow it up in half an hour with cookies and ice cream. But that's what I find myself doing. The chemo seems to have glazed over my rational mind to the point where I don't really care.

My afternoon nap beckons even though it's only 1:00. I look forward to sleep so much these days. It used to be that I'd lie awake at night with thoughts crowding my mind like cars on a highway at rush hour. Now I go upstairs and sink my body down into the cool sheets, claiming sleep, no longer waiting restlessly for it to claim me. This is so new to me. But I'm so eternally tired, what else can I do but lie down and give in to it? I wonder if this is what death is going to be like: sneaking up on me, wearing me out until I just lie down and surrender.

Friday March 15

I'm sitting on the loveseat in the family room with Sasha on my lap, a warm bundle of black fur, her nose pressed lightly against the inside of my knee. The dishwasher churns in the kitchen. Minnie sits on the other sofa, daintily licking her soft gray and white fur. There's nowhere that I have to go, nowhere to be. Just here, safe, healing. Slowly, slowly, healing.

I've been reading all morning. First, at the kitchen table with my breakfast, then on the sofa with Minnie beside me. Now I bask in the very deep pleasure of an afternoon alone. Time stretches before me and I'm safe in its magnificent embrace. Nothing seems impossible in this lazy afternoon light. Nothing. I will have the larger Quiet Room and it will be painted teal and aqua. I will have time to dance, to do yoga, to dream, to create, to write. I will have the time and space in my life to be who I am- no more, no less- just who I am.

Tuesday March 19

About a year ago my friend JoAnn and I started having marathon stamping-talking-creating sessions a few times each month. We were known to start in the morning and still be "playing" at my kitchen table when Jeff came home from work.

Today, however, after just two hours, I put my stamps down and simply sit watching her make a few more cards. She gently asks if I'm tired. Reluctantly, I nod. We put everything away and she leaves with a hug and a promise to call me.

The lack of energy in my body is so discouraging. It's been like this all week. I don't see how women work through these chemo treatments. I feel like some vague shadow of my former self. I can remember in my mind how I used to be. JoAnn and I could stamp all day and into the night, and I'd still have energy left to make supper, write a few emails, and enjoy making love with my husband before I closed my eyes for sleep. My mind remembers this about me, but my body does not.

Thursday March 21

More reading. More napping. More television. Today Rosie O'Donnell is interviewing Kathy Lee Gifford. She's telling Rosie about a friend who lost her husband in one of the Twin Towers on September 11. At the man's funeral, his wife wasn't weeping like everyone else; she was actually glowing. Kathy Lee says you can recognize people who are being supported in prayer because it looks like they're walking in a state of grace, like her friend was that day.

My heart sits up at attention. That is exactly how I felt those first few months after my breast cancer diagnosis. *Walking in a state of grace.* I still feel that way, just not as intensely now. Well, maybe that's not quite true. It's just that yesterday was really hard. I was lethargic from the chemo, and discouraged because of the back and leg pain from the Neupogen. Usually I do feel strongly held in the arms of grace, and I am sure it's because so many people are praying for me.

I smile to myself and change channels, grateful for this gentle reminder of grace which has come to me unexpectedly in the guise of a TV talk show.

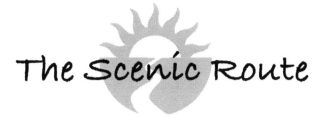

CHAPTER SIXTEEN

The Scenic Route

The longest journey is the journey inward.

— *Dag Hammarskjold*

Sunday March 24

The house is quiet and peaceful in the early morning light. Everyone else is still asleep. I breathe deeply into the silence of my new Quiet Room space, and my heart feels hopeful.

Friday night Jeffrey helped Jeff take apart the bunk beds and then moved the rest of the furniture downstairs. Yesterday Jeff finished painting the room for me. Three of the walls are a dark, exotic shade of teal, and the fourth is a soft aqua. Merri's friend Ryan is visiting this weekend, so he helped Jeff move my loveseat, desk, art table and bookcase into the room. I've hung white eyelet lace curtains at the window; they look just right against the dark teal wall. All that I need now is another long art table, and a small table to place under the window as an altar. I'm going to move my art supplies and books and everything else in here a little bit at a time this week, as I can.

Last night I had another bout of feeling sorry for myself. I cried when we got home from taking Merri and Ryan to dinner, because all I could do was sit in bed and watch TV. I desperately wanted to be in my new Quiet Room, moving things in, setting things up, putting things away. But I'm limited these days. Feeling disabled because of the sore arm, the puffy waxy eyelids, the hemorrhoids, the yeast infection and…. Oh wow, listen to me. I sound… I *feel*… like an old, old woman. I'm too young to have even one of these ailments, much less all of them at once. I know in my head that it's all from the chemo and that it won't last. None of it will last. But living in the midst of my body's unexpected mayhem, it's hard to remember that.

One good thing is that my taste buds are back to normal again. I don't have to eat tons of sugary, fatty food to get the metallic taste out of my mouth. Only one more week until I get chemo-zapped again. I'm not looking forward to it.

Tonight in bed, I lie on my back and once again imagine that loving Presence sitting beside me, stroking my head, listening to me. I name the things I'm grateful for, and what I need forgiveness for. I name what I need, then say the names of others who need healing and peace as well. This is becoming a welcome nightly ritual. A ritual full of comfort, grace and healing.

Tuesday March 26

My new Quiet Room looks wonderful! The art tables are set up and organized; everything is within easy reach. I'm longing to get messy, to create some more of those collages using acrylic paints and handmade paper. It feels so good to have some energy again, to feel more like doing something instead of lying in bed all day flipping channels with the remote control.

As I organize the rest of the space, I find boxes of my writing files in the back of the closet, where they landed when we moved here because I had no time to look at them. Short stories. Essays. Notes for novels in bright colored ink. Now as I gaze at the notebooks and files scattered on the honey-colored carpet, I wonder if I'll ever write seriously again. I recall the passion I once had for writing, remember how I *needed* to write, and how it fed me. Will I ever get to that place again?

Five days until my next chemo treatment. Oh, I don't even want to think about it, particularly the horrid feeling in my mouth and stomach that starts before I even leave the building. Last time, Elly brought me a tuna sandwich on wheat bread in one of those plastic containers from the deli, and now just the thought of a sandwich or plastic container makes me nauseous. I think on Monday I'll have a late breakfast and simply avoid eating lunch during the treatment.

My left eye is itchy and watery and I have to keep dabbing at it with a tissue even though my inclination is to rub it fiercely. I thought I had pink eye yesterday and I called Dr. Morganstern, but he said it's most likely from the chemo and he'll look at it on Monday.

Let's see, what else is wrong with me? My eyelashes have thinned into nonexistence. I still have these annoying hemorrhoids and slight burning/itching feeling in my vaginal area. I'm tired, but not as much as I was last week. Am trying to pace myself as far as working on the Quiet Room is concerned, monitoring fatigue as well as my left arm. There is so much to remember now in order to take care of myself, and most of the time even the thinking is exhausting.

This afternoon the unemployment office calls to tell me that my claim has been denied. I keep thinking there must be a mistake, but the woman assures me it's true. I hang up the phone and panic moves in like an unwelcome, overbearing guest. I pace back and forth in the bedroom, then finally lie down and sob until I can hardly breathe, gulping air frantically.

When the tears subside, I call Jeff who assures me that everything is going to be all right. He tells me not to worry. If all else fails, he will pay my bills until I can go back to work, reminding me that we have extra money in the budget now that we are no longer paying child support for Merri. His calm, familiar voice steadies me. Instead of crying again, I allow a feeling of extraordinary gratitude to wash through me. Gratitude for everything- God's gracious timing, Jeff's gorgeous generosity, the certainty of his love for me.

All shall be well and all shall be well and all manner of thing shall be well. This used to be simply a sentence that resonated with me. Now it is becoming the pattern for my journey.

Wednesday March 27

I'm reading a book called *Learning To Fall,* a series of essays by Philip Simmons who is dying of Hodgkin's Disease. I was afraid it was going to be depressing but it isn't. It's about joy, about life and the living of it, about life's imperfections and beauty even in the midst of suffering. I'm overwhelmed with the sheer perfection of truth and wisdom packed into this one slim volume.

When I started reading it, I wondered if I was crazy to be reading a book by and about a man who is dying. But I have stopped the fearful voices in my head that would shield me from anything to do with the D word. This book is an affirmation of life and living, not a sad tale about dying.

Once in a while, though, I do think of it. Death. What if the cancer returns and I have to go through this all over again? What if it metastasizes and gets out of control, takes over my body?

There are so many *what ifs* in my life now. And somehow I have to content myself with the knowledge that I have no answers….that there are no guarantees. None. From my doctors, from God, from anyone. I have to become comfortable with the assumption that I'm going to live a long and healthy life. I must focus on that and believe it, otherwise the worry and fear will always gain the upper hand.

Saturday March 30

This is the best day I've had in a long time. I spend several hours in my Quiet Room, finishing up some collage pieces that have been sitting on the table for weeks.

Joe drives Mom up for a visit and we meet for lunch at Bertucci's. The drive alone takes six hours out of his day whenever he does this and I am enormously grateful for this generous gift of time and presence, family and laughter. The sky may be gray and dreary, but the sun is shining in my soul.

Jeff and I make love tonight for the first time in weeks. I weep with relief briefly afterwards while he holds me. I've been longing so much for this closeness, this intimacy, but chemo exhaustion has made it impossible.

Sleep claims me once again, deep and insistent. I dream that I'm back at the theatre, walking down a wide, light-filled lobby. There are floor-to-ceiling glass windows on my right, and I'm wearing a bright red short-sleeved dress with a wide swinging skirt. I feel light and happy. There are lots of theatre people milling around, and Jeff is beside me. There are four words that are crystal clear in my mind as we walk down the lobby. *Every moment is precious.*

I awaken with this sentence permanently etched in my mind, and claim it as my personal mantra.

Every moment is precious.

Every **moment** is precious.

Every moment **is** precious.

Every moment is **precious**.

Sunday March 31

I've always had a strange fondness for naming the inanimate objects in my life. Today I decide to name my wig Gracie, as my life these days feels like one perpetual expression of Grace.

I'm not exactly bald like Kojak; there's still a little "fuzz" left on my head. I didn't expect that. But I'm bald enough to wear Gracie whenever I leave the house. I am focusing on the joy of having straight hair for the first time in my life, although I really do miss my curls. One thing's for sure… I will never EVER take my hair for granted again.

Wednesday April 3

Today I feel like crap. I'm taking the anti-nausea meds like clockwork, as usual, but now I feel actually nauseous, instead of only borderline. I'm not so certain that I won't actually have to throw up. The metallic taste has made a dramatic comeback. Pretty much all I can do is lie in bed with the covers up to my neck. The television is on but I find myself drifting off to sleep during my favorite Tom Cruise movies and *Golden Girls* reruns.

Later in the afternoon I drag myself out of bed to put Connie's meat-loaf in the oven, and to make macaroni and cheese. Going up and down the stairs several times is exhausting. When I finally make it upstairs with my plate of food, I feel my hands and feet become cold and tingly, almost numb. My breathing is labored and blackness starts to close in on me, blackness with some dizzying silver stars around the edges. I quickly set the plate down on the bureau and sit on the edge of the bed for a moment. A wave of concentrated heat passes over me, starting at my head and slowly burning its way down through the rest of my body. My fingers are still tingling and I feel like I'm standing in the center of a blazing campfire. I close my eyes but the room begins to spin crazily so I open them again. I'm terrified. Jeff isn't home from work yet, and I'm wondering if I should call someone to come and be with me. I try to relax, taking some deep breaths. I shakily make my way to the windowseat and open both windows halfway, then lie back down on the bed again. The cool fresh air seems to help. I lie absolutely still for about half an hour before the waves of heat and dizziness subside and I feel a little bit more like myself again.

There were a few minor episodes like this last month, when I felt like I simply had to sit down immediately or I would collapse. This incident was similar, only ten times more intense, combined unjustly with a major hot flash. All I want to do now is curl up in the cool sheets and let the bed hold me for the next four weeks until the chemo is over with for good. My lack of control over my own body is incredibly humiliating and frustrating. This is one reason why I indulge in a weekly manicure: it's one small comfort I can give my body- a consistent and proven comfort. It's the same reason for my monthly massage- one more gift I can give myself that eases my body and restores my sense of control.

Saturday April 6

It's 5:30 when I awaken, alert and hungry. It feels like forever since I've gotten up this early! I eat cereal and a buttered English muffin, then retreat into my Quiet Room and simply sit, looking around in wonder. This space is mine, it's really mine. It's big enough for everything I love to do- reading on the loveseat, writing at the desk, and creating art at the two spacious art tables. Yes, this room is big enough, even for yoga, which I did earlier this week, and for dancing, which I don't have the energy for yet but am fantasizing about nearly every day.

Jeff is paying my bills now because my unemployment claim was denied. It's a bit distressing to be totally dependent on him. Not that he's complaining, because he's not. I'm trying to look at this as one more Gift in the midst of all the turmoil. I'm trying to remember how perfectly timed this is. I'm bringing in no money at the exact same time our child support payments for Merri have stopped. We need the money; we have the money. This makes it easier not to feel guilty about being reliant on Jeff. I simply have to let go of my pride, because what choice do I have? It feels like everything has come into alignment for me, so that I can focus my energies on resting, healing, creating.

Jeff and I make love again late this afternoon, and it is lovely, so lovely. Cuddling in the lazy afternoon sunshine under the sheets, breathing in his clean soapy scent, unbuttoning his yellow shirt, feeling closer to him than ever before. I do love this man- completely, wholly, joyously.

Wednesday April 10

I finally feel good enough to attend another support group meeting. The March meeting took place during the beginning of a chemo cycle and I didn't have the energy to attend. I'm still exhausted today but I stay in bed to conserve my energy. At 4:00 I shower and dress, fill my water bottle and get into the car with my new extra-large fanny pack around my waist. No shoulder purse for me; I still greatly fear lymphedema. Of course, I could carry my purse over my *right* shoulder, but I can't seem to get used to that, so I've opted for the fanny pack.

It feels good to see these familiar faces again in the conference room. The guest speaker tonight is a nurse from Lahey, and she does an excellent presentation on lymphedema- what it is, what causes it, and steps to take to prevent it. I realize during the course of the evening that I've been better prepared for this than most of the others, and I'm grateful. But the whole topic is downright scary. I detest the fear that is building inside of me. Fear and worry. Do I want to travel by plane again? Because if I do, I might need to wear a pressure sleeve since flying is yet another thing that induces lymphedema.

I try to shake some of this anxiety off as I walk slowly to my car when the meeting is over, but it remains rooted in my body and mind. I don't want a huge swollen arm on top of everything else. It's bad enough that I can't wear my wedding ring anymore because of the slight swelling in my fingers and hand.

Friday April 12

I scuffle downstairs in sweatpants and an old t-shirt to answer the doorbell, wondering who could be here this early in the morning. The delivery woman standing on the porch holds a huge bouquet of beautiful spring flowers in lovely shades of lavender, rose, soft yellow and white. I thank her and carry the flowers inside, opening the card in the kitchen. *We wish you health and happiness…….. and your computer is still waiting! Love from your theatre family.* My eyes blur with tears as I fill my largest crystal vase with this gorgeous reminder of spring, this tender reminder that I am missed, that I am loved.

Saturday April 13

I wake up very early this morning and go to my Quiet Room, reading on the loveseat with Sasha curled on my lap for a good long time. When I tire of sitting, I do a few minutes of yoga stretches, then sit and meditate, breathing deeply and using the phrase *Every moment is precious.* I love this mantra, and feel certain of its power to carry over into my everyday life if I simply breathe it in enough during morning meditation.

Amanda calls this morning. She asks how I am, but I'm unsure how much she really wants to know so I tell her I'm fine. Jeff gets on the extension and we listen to her chatter happily about her adventures. Her excitement lights up the telephone wires from Pennsylvania to Beverly. It's so good to hear her voice. I also realize that I'm a little envious of her youth and health and independence. I wish I had the freedom that involves getting in a car and driving somewhere with someone you love for the sheer fun of it.

Later today I take part in a three hour art class at a nearby stamp store. This is so much fun, playing with colors, experimenting with some new kinds of paint. The teacher is a well-known paper and fabric artist. As we create, she mentions that her husband doesn't travel with her anymore because he has Hodgkin's Disease. He stays home and helps her run the business from there. Her love for him is evident from the glow on her face when she speaks of their life in the southwest. I listen with interest, up to my elbows in paint and paper. I'm acutely aware that she's talking about cancer. Is it simply everywhere? Can I not get away from it, even for an afternoon?

I haven't been to this stamp store since my diagnosis, and the owner does a double-take when she sees me by the register at the end of the class. She is delighted with my new hairstyle. I debate whether to tell her that this is a wig and why I'm wearing it, but decide to simply thank her. I'm secretly thrilled. Obviously I don't look *so* bad or she would guess right away that I've been sick. Let her think I got my hair straightened and colored. So what?

Monday April 15

Today is difficult. The fatigue from the third treatment has lasted longer than from the first two treatments. It's difficult to accept that my old energy is no longer a part of me. There's so much I want to *do* today, but all I have energy for is sitting still and reading. So that is what I do. I try to be gentle with myself, to remind myself exactly what my body is dealing with here. Yet this is easier said than done. My tendency has always been to do, do, do…go, go, go….. and here I am now, stuck in neutral. I have to remind myself over and over that being still is a fundamental part of the healing process, that the hours of reading and napping are feeding my body and soul in a way that is crucial to my recovery.

I climb into bed before 9:00 tonight, and within ten minutes of closing my eyes, I feel the beginnings of a very bad headache. I haven't had one in several months, and the strangeness of it scares me. I'm immediately wide-awake and alert, my heart pounding in my chest. The headache brings with it a tangible fear.

Ordinarily I would go to the bathroom, flick on the light, swallow some ibuprofen with water and head back to the shelter of sleep. But now, with the words *breast cancer* shading everything that happens to me, I find myself panicking in the darkness, certain that the cancer has metastasized to my brain, certain that I have a brain tumor. My mind spins these thoughts round and round until they are whirling out of control. Should I call the doctor? But which doctor should I call? Should I call now or should I wait until morning? Maybe I should just go right now to the Emergency Room. Do people actually *go* to the Emergency Room for headaches?

There is some level of sanity left in my muddled brain, because I'm aware of the craziness of my thoughts, and in this awareness I resolve to calm down. I take a few deep breaths, rub my head, look fear in the face and decide to take action. I get up and look at myself in the bathroom mirror. I look okay, in spite of the fact that my hair is gone, my eyebrows are ragged, and there are dark shadows under my eyes. I whisper *I love you* to the face in the mirror, fill a clear blue glass with water, feel its coolness sliding down my throat along with three small ibuprofen pills. I murmur comforting words to myself on the way back to bed, like a mother soothing a crying child. *There, there. You're going to be okay. The medicine will start to work in a few minutes.*

And indeed, it does.

Tuesday April 16

I open the mail to find a Thinking of You card from someone I worked with several years ago, someone who was fired because she was stealing money from the company. It was almost impossible to believe, but I was one of the managers there at the time and I actually saw visible proof that she had done this. I look at the card several times this afternoon, note the familiar flowery handwriting, read her words of kindness, and wonder if I should respond to her. We haven't spoken since the day she was escorted from the building. The whole thing is still somewhat incomprehensible to me. She was one of the best bosses I've ever had: consistently fair, kind, fun, and loyal to her employees. We had worked together closely for a few years and yet there was no closure when she left. Her leaving felt like betrayal and abandonment; I don't believe I've ever forgiven her. Perhaps now would be a good time to begin that process.

I've learned a lot about forgiveness over the last eleven years with Jeff and his children. My mother keeps pushing me to forgive Amanda and Jeffrey, but I think she's got it all wrong. I have totally forgiven them for rejecting my love over and over again. They were children; it was never their fault that they felt pulled in different directions. It still hurts when I think of those days, but that is simply the part of me that's always had a hard time with rejection. I know that they never meant to hurt me. They were caught in a bizarre whirlwind of being made to choose between their mother and me, and of course they chose her. They could have had both of us, if their mother could have accepted me and not put them in the middle, but they were not allowed this. So my mother is wrong. It is neither Amanda or Jeffrey whom I need to forgive. It is their mother.

And what about *me*? Have I ever forgiven *myself* for not being able to love Amanda and Jeffrey unconditionally? Have I forgiven myself for not living up to my own impossibly high standards of being a stepmother? For not being able to keep our stepfamily together the way I deeply wanted to? I don't think I have consciously been able to forgive myself for these self-defined "failures," yet I have the feeling that therein lies the key to more inner healing for me.

It's always been so difficult to forgive myself. And this becomes just one more way of being hard on myself, one more way of labeling myself a failure. I need to find a way to stop doing this.

Jeff is very good at forgiveness. He hardly knows the meaning of holding a grudge. Sometimes, when I'm really down on myself, I wonder what he sees in me, wonder if he is secretly disappointed in me because I wasn't the best stepmother, and now I've got breast cancer, of all things.

But the other night at dinner, he leaned across the table, took my hand in his and told me *I'd not have life without you in it.* My heart caught in my throat as he said this, and I had to look away. Jeff doesn't usually express his feelings with words, so this was especially powerful. There are tears in my eyes even now, remembering it. What if I do die from breast cancer and he has to live without me? I know it's only a slight possibility, but even the smallest possibility of *this* sort is cause for deep reflection.

And the other thought that is taking up major space in my head is this: what would *my* life be like without *him* in it? It seems that facing my own mortality makes others' seem equally as fragile, especially those I love the most

CHAPTER SEVENTEEN

Souvenirs to Take Home

All changes, even the most longed for, have their melancholy;
for what we leave behind us is a part of ourselves;
we must die to one life before we can enter another.
— Anatole France

Wednesday April 17

I feel like I've been unearthing parts of myself in a psycho-archeo-logical dig. There are writing files and pages of half-finished stories, novels and essays strewn all over my Quiet Room floor. Part of me is eager to look through them, delve into them like a swimmer submerging herself in warm tranquil waters. But another part of me is a little anxious about what I'll find, and won't allow myself to look. In the course of the day, I go to the doorway of the room several times, pause to survey the scene, then walk quickly past. It feels like I'm doing a strange dance with my Writing Self.

It is late afternoon by the time I finally stop the dance. I step into the

Quiet Room and sit down in the middle of the floor. It's been years since I wrote or looked at any of this, and I find myself drawn in immediately. There are short stories, several folders of essays, a young adult novel, scraps and bits of dialog and character sketches which might find their way to novels one day.

Yes, these are my words. Yes, this is me leaping off of these pages, embedded in these stories, hidden in these paragraphs. I remember writing every word. Reading all of this is like coming home somehow, coming home to myself. It's like finding a part of myself that I'd lost along the way. Now I sit here and savor the tender beginnings that show potential (and some that don't), the stories that are complete, the essays that show deep thought and wisdom.

After a few hours I reluctantly stand, stretch, and leave the room, heading for the kitchen to make supper. Jeff will be hungry when he gets home from work. I am not hungry, however. I find that I'm full, completely full to the brim with the words I have written, with the stories and characters that I alone have created. I set the table, turn on the oven, prepare the salmon. But I'm operating on remote control. I'm dazed with this new awareness: my writing is very *very* good.

And I am left with a resounding, awesome yet terrifying question— *What do I do with this gift?* For surely it is a gift. I almost wrote *What do I do with this gift that I wasted?* But no, I'm being too hard on myself. It hasn't been wasted, just tucked away into a corner of my soul where it's been resting, waiting for me to revive it, welcome it back into my life. But how and when and where exactly do I start? There is so much there just waiting for some loving attention.

One of my current affirmations that I hear and repeat every day on the tape is *I am finding my way to what is next.* I didn't know exactly what I meant when I wrote it, but now it's becoming clearer.

It's very silly, I know, but I'm worried that I won't get everything done….. and I still have ten weeks left of my time off. I'm trying to counteract this worry by reminding myself that by going back to work part time instead of full time, I'll be creating time and space in my life for the things that fill me with life and joy: my writing and my art.

Jeff tells me tonight that he's going to take Monday off and come with me to my last chemo treatment. I protest but he insists and I don't argue again. It's our seventh anniversary and it will be comforting to have him there.

Thursday April 18

I shrug into the ugly gray hospital gown with the tiny checkered print. It's time for my three month post-surgery check-up with Dr. Karp. Has it really only been three months? It feels more like three years.

I notice how relieved I am to see him again. He is a connection to the trauma of my diagnosis and two surgeries. He is my connection to the beginning of this journey, and even though he didn't experience it in a similar fashion, it's like we've survived some major disaster together, and I feel deeply attached to him because of it.

My internet search for surgical caps with carp on them has been successful, and there are three of them in my tote bag which is resting against the gray and blue metal chair. It turns out that carp are a domesticated kind of fish otherwise known as koi. Who knew?

I want to give the caps to him today, but I feel incredibly nervous about it. I know that this isn't an ordinary gift, although I have absolutely no idea if other women even *think* of giving presents to their doctors. I'm anxious because I don't know if giving a doctor a gift like this is stepping across some unwritten boundary. My shyness surfaces and I feel like a twelve year old with a crush on her favorite teacher, even though in reality I'm a happily married forty-six year old woman who has just faced cancer with the fierce determination of a lion tamer facing the lion.

I spend the rest of the day berating myself because I chickened out after having gone to all the trouble of having the caps made for him. I write about it in my daily email to Dawn and she replies immediately, telling me that I *have* to give Dr. Karp those caps, no matter what. She understands my shyness but reassures me that he'll love the gift, reiterates that she's certain he will appreciate them. I breathe a sigh of relief when I read her reply.

I know! I can give the caps to Mary on Monday when I see her at my last chemo. She sees Dr. Karp every day; she can deliver them to him for me. I've already decided to give Ellie and Dr. Morganstern boxes of my handmade note cards as "Celebration-Of-My-Last-Chemo" gifts; I will give a Celebration gift to Dr. Karp as well. Yes. This feels absolutely right to me.

Sunday April 21

Tonight Jeff and I head for a nice seafood restaurant in Essex, and eat our anniversary dinner sitting side by side, looking across the river. It's a beautiful evening, the setting sun is painting the sky with sweet strokes of golden rose, and a soft breeze cools my skin. As I lean against Jeff and he kisses my forehead, I realize once again how blessed and privileged I am to have him beside me on this journey.

Later, getting ready for bed, I find myself thinking about tomorrow. *Just the thought* of sitting in that big gray chair with the bags on the pole beside me is actually enough to make me feel a little bit nauseous. The awful metallic taste makes a reappearance in my mouth as I simply *think* about the blood work, the waiting room, the sunroom, the chair, Ellie. No one is ever going to tell me again that there's no mind-body connection! I haven't had this nasty taste in my mouth for over a week, so I know it's all in my mind. I try doing some visualization exercises, focusing on the stories I'm going to tell Ellie, the gifts I'm giving. This eases the nausea somewhat, and the harsh taste in my mouth lessens but remains.

Monday April 22

The metallic sensation in my mouth is stronger and more horrible than ever this morning. There is no getting rid of it, no matter how many distracting visualizations I try to do. I resign myself to it with a deep sigh, and breathe deeply through the entire morning instead of holding my breath like I want to.

Mary, the Lahey clinical trial assistant, meets me in the waiting room with a hug and news of her med school exams. She chatters non-stop and I'm grateful for the beautiful distraction. I give her a box of my handmade note cards, and allow myself to fully savor the delight of her response. Then I give her the bag of surgical caps for Dr. Karp. She takes them out of the bag and with genuine excitement lacing her voice, tells me over and over that he'll love them. I feel elated and relieved and deeply satisfied with her response. She hugs me again as Ellie comes to the front desk and calls my name. I wonder if I will ever see Mary again. I wonder if she will ever know how truly healing her presence in my life has been these past few months.

I enjoy the pleasure of giving the cards to Ellie, who expresses joyful surprise at the unexpected gift. We entertain each other with tales of Easter dinners gone awry as the jewel-toned drugs drip their way steadily into my veins. As Jeff and I are leaving, I give her Dr. Morganstern's box of cards and she promises to give them to him tomorrow. Ellie hugs me tightly. Usually I dissolve into tears at good-byes like this, but…. have I ever experienced a good-bye like this one? I'm aware of our connection, aware that I'll miss her sunny smile, our easy conversation. But I'm also aware that I can't get out of here quickly enough. I never want to see this place again.

At home, I immediately put on my nightgown and get into bed even though it's only 2:00. I know what's coming; there's no sense avoiding it by running around doing errands and checking email like I did that first time. I decide to lie still and not fight it. I'm incredibly grateful and relieved that the treatments are over. I have sat in that huge recliner in the light-filled "sun room" for the last time. A few more weeks of physical wretchedness and I'll be back on the road to Real Healing.

Before I drift off into this chemical-induced sleep, I check my voice-mail messages and listen with joy to Dr. Karp's voice telling me he's just received the surgical caps from Mary and that he is absolutely *blown away*. This is the very best, most thoughtful gift he has ever received, he tells me, and I can hear the genuine pleasure in his voice. I'm imagining him still holding the caps in his hand as he's talking on the phone, and I smile with deep satisfaction. He likes the gift. I have crossed no obscure boundary. The gift has given joy and delight to someone who has given me healing and another chance at life. I close my eyes and allow sleep to claim me. All is well.

Saturday April 27

This has been the longest week of my life, waiting for the nausea to subside and the metallic taste in my mouth to disappear (it still hasn't, quite).

I feel more like *me* today and that feels decidedly good. I have actually gotten out of bed, taken a warm bath, and am sitting at my desk, writing. The window beside me is open, a gentle breeze flutters the white curtains. There are several art projects spread out on the worktables behind me, and I'm aware of their presence there, awaiting my attention.

It feels so good to be creating all of this art. Not just good, but incredibly abundant. Almost decadent. Like I'm rich, sated, full, internally wealthy beyond my wildest dreams. It's not about money, it's about creating art from the depths of my soul.

Sleep eludes me tonight so I sit up for a few hours reading more of the writing I did years ago. Some of the writing exercises are forced, but some of it (especially the fiction) is actually very good. I stare into space for a while after I put down the notebook, keenly aware of my body and mind finally aligning for sleep.

Monday April 29

It's a dreary afternoon splashed with rain, but please take note- I'm *not* watching TV or lying in bed with the covers drawn up to my neck. I'm sitting at a *Barnes and Noble* bookstore, looking at writing magazines and indulging in a mocha coconut coffee drink that tastes divine.

The people around me are sipping various forms of caffeine, deeply engrossed in a variety of conversations, or standing in the aisles leafing through books. It occurs to me that not one of them would look at me and think anything other than the fact that I'm a 40-something woman reading a magazine. This realization has a lovely, normalizing effect on me. I decide to buy two of the magazines spread out on the table before me. Why the heck not? I am a writer.

I'm filled with gratitude for being able to devote these months to my healing, my art, my writing. It's like the breast cancer diagnosis (and the subsequent time off), has given me a respite from who I thought I was. It's like I've been given a lift out of a rut that I didn't even know I was in.

I feel like I'm being given an intimate, valuable gift: the perspective that this time off is a resting place, an oasis located between *Who I Was* and *Who I'm Going To Be*. I am inhabiting a sanctuary on a journey between my self-perceived, self-defined concept of myself as failure (as a stepmother mostly), and my new self-declared concept of myself as success (as artist and writer and survivor of a deadly disease). I'm like an insect, quiescent in my cocoon (the haven that is allowing me to remember who I am at my deepest core) before I burst forth with rainbows of color and my wings spread wide.

I feel like there is no end to the possibilities before me. No end to what I can create, what I will create. No end to the inner discoveries that await me.

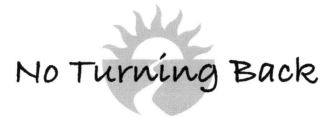

CHAPTER EIGHTEEN

No Turning Back

I am not afraid of storms, for I'm learning how to sail my ship.
— *Louisa May Alcott*

Wednesday May 8

I've outgrown a few of the daily affirmations that I began using in February so I'm rewriting them. One that came to me last night is *I face my fears with courage and they turn to love.*

I've been noticing how prevalent fear is in my life these days, how it controls many of my moment-to-moment decisions. The other morning I heard Jeff's mom talking with Joe, our new stage manager at the theatre. I could hear them in the kitchen and I thought I'd just go in and introduce myself. That's when my fear set in. *Fear of what?* Of being judged by him? Of him not liking me? Of having to discuss why I'm currently not at the theatre? Of having to explain why I'm wearing a wig? A little bit of each?

I had to take myself by the hand and talk gently to my inner self, like I would talk to a small child afraid of walking into the classroom on the first day of school. I reminded myself gently that I'd had enough courage to face breast cancer, two surgeries, chemotherapy, and being bald, so perhaps I had enough courage to introduce myself to this new person. So I did. And of course, everything was all right. Joe didn't judge me and I didn't need to mention the cancer once.

Now I'm noticing some fear around going to the *Ragtime* dress rehearsal on Monday night. It takes me by surprise as I ordinarily love going to dress rehearsals. I spend some time thinking about what is making me fearful. I know I'll be receiving a lot of focused attention from the people I know who'll be there. Perhaps I'm afraid of the energy I'll expend answering every single person who asks me how I'm doing. I wonder how people will react to seeing me again. Perhaps I'm also afraid of the onslaught of emotion I will feel at being there again in my second home, after so many months away.

I don't want fear to keep me away from people and places that I love so dearly. I am repeating this new affirmation like a mantra today. *I face my fears with courage and they turn to love.*

I'm so grateful for the time and space to be discovering these things about myself. I'm learning to take life slowly and on its own terms; to be trusting of the process instead of trying to control it. I'm hoping that when I go back to work I'll be able to maintain this new sense of Self that I didn't have before. This time off has allowed me the privilege of self-discovery, a blessing that is opening many new roads to me.

Thursday May 9

Tonight is the last support group meeting in Burlington. I take several handmade bookmarks with me to give to the women at the meeting. The backgrounds are various shades of pink pigment ink sponged onto white cardstock. The words COURAGE, STRENGTH, and HOPE are stamped on each bookmark along with the breast cancer ribbon which is encircled with flowers that I shaded in with bright colored pencils. I tied purple and blue yarn tassels through the hole in the top of each one. The women are oohing and ahhing as they each take one from the pile I've placed in the center of the table, and this makes me feel content, happy.

Friday May 10

The after-effects of the cancer are always right here, staring me in the face. I don't think they'll ever really disappear. Every day there's something that I have to remember or worry over. Is that bag of birdseed too heavy for me to pick up? Should I carry the laundry basket upstairs or ask Jeff to do it? Is my arm okay? What's that bump on my leg? Has this bruise on my hip been there more than a week? Did the chemotherapy kill all of the cancer or are there still some stray cells roaming through my body, ready to explode at the smallest sign of stress, the slightest provocation?

And then there's sex. More often than not I just don't feel like making love. I know many of the reasons are physical ones: menopause, fatigue and the chemotherapy drugs. But I also know that some of the reasons are emotional ones, that I just don't feel very sexual these days. And who could blame me, really? I have no hair; there are dark shadows under my eyes and I feel tired all of the time. More people have looked at my bare breasts in the last six months than in the entire 45 years of my existence. And when I think about the numbers of well-intentioned medical professionals who've poked and prodded my body in various places, and stuck countless needles in my arm and hand, well…. it's mighty difficult to feel sexy.

When I'm at my most insecure, I wonder if Jeff is just saying he doesn't mind all these changes simply because he knows it's the right thing to say. But I can't hold onto that particular insecurity; I simply don't have the energy for it. I have to trust that he is sincere and truthful, as he has been for the eleven years I've known and loved him.

This afternoon I go into the Radiation Department at Lahey for my simulation, where the technicians will measure my breast and mark it for accurate radiation treatments. I lie flat on my back for over an hour on a narrow steel table, my hospital gown open with my left breast hanging out while four people scurry back and forth between the small back room and the large room I'm in. There are two technicians here with Dr. Girshovich, and a very handsome man who is from the Physics Department.

I had no idea that hospitals even *had* Physics Departments, much less that it would be involved in my radiation treatments. Having struggled with this particular subject in high school and college, I find it ironic that Physics is to be an integral part of my therapy. The Physics Specialist measures my left breast from every conceivable angle with several cold metal instruments. He is intently focused on his work, jots down notes on a clipboard from time to time, confers with the doctor about the best places for the radiation markers. I only have a vague, rudimentary understanding of what they're doing, although I can see graphs and calculations flashing on a screen over in the corner of the room. I really don't want to know any more. My job is to lie still with my left arm stretched over my head (uncomfortable as that is) and trust these four people with the next segment of my healing.

The two technicians are quite different in appearance. Val is thin and angular with long straight pale blonde hair. She seems focused on the work at hand rather than on me. Linda is shorter and a little rounder with short brown hair and a smile that warms me inside and out. She's the one who welcomed me into the Simulation Room, got me settled on the table and has already discovered that I work at the theatre, that I'm an artist. There is something about her, some irrepressible kindness that makes me feel safe. I feel like she really *sees* me. It's easy to lie back and trust that everything will continue to be well, because she is here looking out for me.

An hour goes by and Val mentions that Linda has to leave a little early because of a doctor's appointment. Panic sets in. I don't want her to leave, but it's currently not in my power to protest.

They're drawing large crosses and X's on my breast with a purple Sharpie pen as if I were a poster board. I find this amusing also. With such sophisticated medical technology at our disposal, I'd expect them to be using a more advanced instrument. But no, they're using a marker that anyone can buy at WalMart.

Linda is still here even though it's past 3:00. When I ask her why, she cheerfully tells me that her doctor won't mind if she's a little late. Genuine tears come to my eyes as a river of gratitude flows into my heart. She isn't going to leave me. Somehow she knows that I feel connected to her and she's going to stay with me until this strange procedure is over. I thank her as best I can from flat on the table, and wonder if she can possibly know the depth of my gratitude.

Half an hour later, Val shows me a small "gun" and tells me she's going to make four permanent tiny tattoo marks on my breast. These marks will be what they use to line up the machine that will deliver the radiation treatments to my body, so that the rays will go to the correct area of my breast.

Linda is getting ready to go now, and Val chides her for leaving. It seems that the tattoos will sting a bit when the gun marks me, and Val tells Linda she's sure I'm going to hate her forever for doing it. They're laughing, and I laugh with them, suddenly happy that Val is here. I know now that she has truly seen me because she knew exactly what I was thinking. She tells me that each mark will sting but only for a moment, and she is right. It feels like four quick bee stings, one right after the other. The tattoo marks are a deep indigo, about as big as a pinhead.

I put my bra and shirt back on. I'm so tired right now that the hard metal table appears to be beckoning me to lie down again. I was going to go shopping, buy myself a new rubber stamp and ink pad to reward myself for getting through this. But that isn't going to happen today. I drive home slowly, glad that the next step of the journey is behind me, grateful for the welcoming bed and cozy afghan that await me at home.

Monday May 13

It's only 9 p.m. but I'm bleary-eyed with need of sleep. The *Ragtime* dress rehearsal is about to begin and I've somehow managed to get myself to the theatre just in time. This is our first musical this season and I've missed being part of the box office madness that precedes our first show. I missed *Show and Tell* last month, when the production staff talks about the set design, the costumes, the special effects. I missed the *Meet and Greet* two weeks ago when theatre staff gets to meet the cast before they start rehearsals. I missed the *Designers Run-Through* last week, the first beginning-to-end performance that staff is invited to before they move into the theatre for tech rehearsals. And I've missed hearing the music floating from the stage into the lobby and over to the box office.

But I'm here now and it feels perfectly wonderful to step through the big red doors into the magic that is our theatre. At first I feel slightly disoriented because I haven't been here for so long. But then Joan and Jocelyn are here, welcoming me with warm hugs that ground me into how truly connected I am in spite of everything. I wave to a few of the head ushers and other staff members who seem pleased to see me. I sigh with pleasure and sink deeper into the red cushioned seat, giving myself over to the enchant-ment of the story, the music, the characters on our circular stage.

Towards the end, one of the female characters sings a song called *Back to Before* and I catch my breath when I hear the words. She sings of how she has changed and grown since her husband left on his expedition to the North Pole, how things outside of her have changed as well. She may as well be sing-ing about me in that clear strong soprano voice. I can never go back to how my life was before breast cancer.

My own internal and external worlds have changed incredibly; both look considerably different to me now and I know they always will. My life will never be the same again. And the thing is, I don't want it to be the same. I don't want to go back to the way I was before. As difficult as most of these inner and outer changes are, I find that I am now usually able to embrace them (and myself) with humility and grace.

CHAPTER NINETEEN

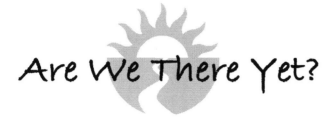

Are We There Yet?

Patience is power.
With time and patience the mulberry leaf becomes silk.

— Chinese Proverb

Wednesday May 15

I take off my t-shirt and bra in one of the dressing rooms in the back of the radiation clinic, and put on the blue hospital gown. In the treatment room I settle myself on yet another narrow metal table. It takes Linda and Val longer to get me "lined up" than to do the actual treatment. They spend several minutes shifting my body around on the table: a slight push here, a soft pull there. I try to cooperate but they tell me not to, so I breathe deeply and consciously relax my muscles, allowing them easier access to manipulate my body into proper alignment.

Before she leaves the room to activate the radiation, Linda turns off the lights and I find that I'm staring at the most beautiful image on the ceiling.

Someone has taken a gorgeous photograph of a winding path covered with red and yellow tulips. The sky is clear blue and there is a hint of a brook in the background. The photo has been blown up to cover the length and width of several ceiling tiles. There are lights behind it so when the room is dark, it seems to be lit from within, beckoning me into it. When Linda tells me not to move, it's easy because I'm focusing on this beautiful image. It warms and relaxes me, making me smile from the inside out. Another gift.

A loud mechanical sound drones on for thirty seconds, stops, then sounds again. Linda and Val come back into the room, flipping on the lights. That's it?

That's it. I swing my legs off the table, covering myself with the flimsy blue gown. This wasn't so bad. I only have to do this 41 more times and I'll be done. I push that thought aside, trying not to think too far ahead or I'll never get through this. One day at a time…. this has to be my mantra during this round of the treatments. One day…. one radiation dose… at a time.

I go to the mall and buy five extra large short-sleeved men's shirts in bright, vivid colors. It's been suggested that going braless will be easier on the skin of the radiated breast, so I need something to wear over my tank tops and t-shirts.

Friday May 17

The second treatment is exactly the same as the first. While I'm lying on the table, I dissolve into the warm spring scene of tulips and flowers at the park, conveniently located on the ceiling over my head. I pretend I'm walking in this park, running through the tulips. I can feel the warm sun on my back, the vigorous sense of life that rushes through my strong healthy body like the wind.

Once again I'm startled at how simple and fast the procedure is. Strip from the waist up. Put on the gown. Lie on the table. Let Linda and Val push and tug at me until I'm in alignment. Zap. Pause. Zap. Time to go.

Monday May 20

I've been feeling rather restless even though it's my birthday. Maybe because it's such a gorgeous day and I feel a little sorry for myself because I have no energy whatsoever to go outside and enjoy the sunshine. Or maybe it's because I slept longer than I intended to.....again.

I've been having more dreams about going back to work. Perhaps I should go back before July 1. I miss my theatre family more than I ever thought I would, yet the pull to stay home is equally great. This interior tug of war intensifies my restlessness.

I've been having a lot of difficulty getting myself out of bed in the morning. I'm wondering if I'm becoming clinically depressed as a result of the tamoxifen, or the culminating effects of so many months of treatments, or...... what? I wake up most mornings by 8:00 but then I just lie there, sometimes drifting back to sleep, sometimes awake but feeling like my legs are made of lead. This is definitely not like me at all. I wonder if knowing that I have to be at the theatre by 8:30 will make it easier for me to get out of bed in the mornings, if it will ease this slight depression before it begins bearing down harder on me.

Also, my left breast is feeling tender and sore, like when I used to have PMS. Except, of course, that it couldn't possibly be PMS because I'm in menopause and my right breast feels perfectly fine. It's totally annoying, and I know it's from the radiation. They told me this was going to happen and that it's going to feel like this for a long time. Wearing a bra makes it feel better but they told me to go braless as much as possible, so I'm doing that even though it makes me uncomfortable. And as if that weren't enough, my left arm is stiffer and more sore than usual, even though it had been feeling really good for a while.

I suppose all of these things keep adding up, and after a while, the weight of them all presses me into depression.

Jeff and I try to make love again tonight but it's so painful that we have to stop. I'm beyond frustrated and annoyed now; I'm seething with anger. Cancer has taken some things (a perfectly shaped left breast, my hair, my energy, the range of motion in my left arm,) from me these past several months, and I've let go of those things with as much grace as I could muster. However,

159

I'm not going to let the cancer rob me of a pleasurable sex life also. I'm seeing a new gynecologist this week and I'll ask her about this new development. Surely there is *something* that modern science can do for me.

Thursday May 23

I email Suzanne today and ask if I can come back to work, part time only, on June 3 instead of July 1. In an hour I have a happy response from her. *YES! Come back quickly, we need you!* I feel relieved now, lighter, like the depression is waning.

Friday May 24

Dr. Petersen, my new gynecologist, is also a breast cancer survivor. My friend Joan has recommended her to me and I'm thoroughly delighted with the time she takes to get to know me before she examines me. I am on the verge of tears as I explain how painful sex is lately, in spite of the miracle of personal lubricants. She nods with understanding. then prescribes a special cream for me to use, and promises that it's going to get better soon. I breathe in her words like a much-needed hit of oxygen. There are answers, solutions. All I had to do was ask.

Sunday June 2

I'm really looking forward to going back to work tomorrow, but am nervous about the first few minutes: how everyone is going to react, how I'm going to feel, how the new staff will respond to me.

I've always had an aversion to being the focus of everyone's attention, but a lot has happened these last months regarding my self-esteem. I like myself a great deal more than I ever did. I respect myself more. I've had so much time and space to be with myself, to notice myself. I feel like I've fallen in love with myself again.

Looking at what I've gone though in just six months, I admire my strength and courage, my bright spirit, my ability to slow my life down, to allow myself to heal. I know I'm not done yet; I still have six weeks of daily radiation treatments to get through. I still have months of healing from the effects of these treatments. But, as tired as I am these days, I can look back on what is past and know that the worst is over.

Weather permitting, I'm taking a daily walk. Sometimes I do a whole mile; sometimes I do half. It seems to be keeping my energy levels up and I'm glad of that. I feel so much more "normal" when I can walk; anything that helps eliminate the self-definition of "sick" is good for me.

Monday June 3

John and Joan are already in the box office when I arrive, and they welcome me with fervent hugs. Joan has put a large metallic rainbow at my computer station along with a lovely hand-lettered sign that says *WELCOME HOME ANNE!* I'm deeply touched.

The others come in as the clock inches closer to 9:00, and all of the "old timers" express delight and hug me when they notice I'm back. It almost seems like I've never been away.

But then again it feels like I've been away for decades because I've been to another landscape altogether while they've been sitting at the same computers, answering the same phones, selling the same tickets. My *inner* landscape has changed; I can look at this room and these people with gratitude and grace now instead of frustration and annoyance.

John sits with me for a few hours this morning and reviews everything with me. How to log into the computer system, sell a ticket, do a subscriber ticket exchange. I'm impressed by his patience and tenderness with me, as well as the respect that the staff has for him. After thanking him sincerely, I spend the rest of the morning reviewing and deleting my 904 emails. I was surprised to see so many. I'd thought that my email would be stopped while I was gone. Most of the messages are irrelevant now but it's interesting to read the all-staff memos; they make me feel like an integral part of the theatre family again.

At 12:30 I log off, pack up my things and say good-bye. It feels strange to leave at lunchtime and know I'm not coming back until tomorrow. When

I get home after the radiation treatment, I lie down for a few hours and slip into a long blessed nap. Sasha seems especially glad to see me. She joins me on the bed, curled up as close to me as she can get. I'm sure she is wondering what happened to me earlier today. It's been a very long time since I left her for an entire morning!

Monday June 17

The fatigue is overwhelming most of the time now and I hate it. For two weeks I haven't felt like sitting at my art table and playing around with new card designs. My afternoons are totally free, but all I have energy for is reading, watching TV, and sleeping. It's different from the chemo fatigue because at least then I knew that the following week I'd have a little more energy, and then even more energy the week after that. I still have three more weeks of radiation treatments and the physical exhaustion is making me emotionally weary and frustrated.

It feels like the treatments have been going on forever and yet the end is nowhere in sight. I'm so tired of how long it's taking to get to the end. Maybe I'm finally starting to feel angry that this has been happening to me. Not just the breast cancer, but everything connected with it that I have to learn to live with- constant hemorrhoids, no eyelashes, scarce eyebrows, weight gain, fear of lymphedema, and the latest consequence- my ten-times-more-sore-than-PMS left breast. I can't wear a bra, which limits my clothing choices. These petty annoyances that interrupt the continuity and quality of my life don't seem so petty when they've been part of my life for so long.

Thursday June 20

Today I can't stand these feelings of anger and exhaustion any longer. I ask Jeff if we can sit down and talk so I can explain how I'm feeling and why I've been acting so crabby and hateful lately. Everyone has told us how "easy" the radiation treatments are compared to the chemo, but they forgot to mention how drained and exhausted I would feel. One thing I know about myself is that whenever I get tired, my inner fuse grows extremely short.

I've written everything I'm thinking and feeling in a two page letter. He has read the letter and the first thing he mirrors back to me is my fatigue, my frustration, my fear. As soon as I hear him acknowledging these feelings, I begin sobbing with the safety of knowing that I've been truly seen and heard.

When my tears have subsided, we talk quietly for a while about some other issues between us, especially how difficult it is for me to have all of his kids living with us again right now. He tells me he wishes it could be different but he wants to unburden his sister from having to look after Merri, and he feels like Amanda needs a safe place to live for a while. I'm able to listen now, to remember how much I love these compassionate, nurturing traits in him, his capacity for unconditional loving.

Afterwards I sit on the front porch steps for several minutes, just breathing in the sweet night air, letting it calm my mind and spirit, letting it soothe my weary body. I've been meditating like this every day for fifteen minutes and I like how it slows and calms me. It helps me to remember who I am.

Wednesday June 26

My mornings and evenings now are polar opposites. In the morning I feel hopeful, almost normal. In the morning, everything is the same as it Used To Be. But by evening I'm so worn out and bone-weary that everything seems dark and out of focus, like I will never have My Life back.

Of course, this isn't true. I know that in a month I'll feel a tiny bit better, and a month after that even more so. It's just so easy to forget this simple fact when the fatigue sets in.

Monday July 1

The skin on my left breast is peeling and it stings like crazy, feels hot and sore. The nurse has told me to keep it dry and *not* to put hydrocortisone cream on it. So I put a cool wet facecloth against the broken skin. Tonight I feel like I'll jump out of my skin altogether if I don't put something on it to stop the throbbing, so I head for the drugstore at midnight to find a natural cream made with aloe.

Wednesday July 3

Today is my last radiation treatment. It's also my last treatment, period. I wake up with the anticipation of freedom vibrating through my soul.

Val and Linda hug me when I'm ready to leave and I find myself ready to cry. I've seen them every day for almost two months; they've become an integral and expected part of my life. I will miss them. I've packaged up some of my note cards as gifts; their delight feeds my need to give something back to them, these radiation angels who have ministered to me on my journey.

I've heard some women say that they weren't happy when their treatments were over because they felt like they were alone and unsupported after months and months of frequent doctor visits and treatments. I thought I might feel that way too when this day came, but I don't.

I feel an exquisite, profound joy expanding within me as I drive away from the hospital. Tomorrow is the Fourth of July. *Independence* Day! I now have a whole new respect for the word *freedom*.

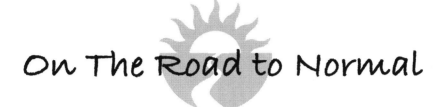

CHAPTER TWENTY

On The Road to Normal

Wheresoever you go, go with all your heart.

— Confucius

Thursday July 4

PERSONAL DECLARATION OF INDEPENDENCE

I, Anne Marie Bennett, have survived six months of breast cancer treatments. The treatments are over now and I am of the firm belief that the cancer is gone, <u>all</u> of it. I hereby declare my independence from the treatments, from the cancer, and from my identity as a patient.

I hereby declare my intention to take care of myself. This is a gift that I give to myself in honor of my inner beauty and strength and power, in honor of my life, in celebration of my triumph over breast cancer, a disease that would have killed me if left unchecked.

From this day forward, my life will be different.

Food will be used for physical nourishment. Meditation will be used for remembering who I am. Life will be savored, moment by moment. Feelings will be fully felt and expressed.

I will be gentle with myself and others. I will practice forgiveness towards myself and others, on a daily and immediate basis. I will continue to let go of the past and look forward to the future with anticipation.

I will remember daily that Life is a precious gift, not to be taken for granted.

I love who I am and who I am becoming.

Sunday July 7

As I meditate, the pure and easy light of morning streams through my open window. I promise myself to continue this practice; it is the key to my healing, to a more joyful life, to living more abundantly, losing weight, and to a whole host of other good things.

Every once in a while I pause to think about what I've just been through and the reality of it brings me up short. I've had breast cancer. Two surgeries, twelve weeks of chemotherapy, forty-two radiation treatments. Holy Mother of God. *Cancer.* The C word. I've known this all along, of course, but suddenly the realization creeps up on me and wham! I am startled into amazement whenever I think of it this way.

I'm also startled by one bitter, raw fact: *it might return.* This truth brings with it a deep, odious, piercing fear, a fear that seems much wider than the world. I have to learn to live with this fear now, but I can't let it control my life. I simply can't. I have to find a way to accept and embrace it without allowing it to control me. Without allowing it to shut me down.

Tuesday July 9

Today I feel like I'm just about at the road that leads to Normal. The skin on my breast doesn't hurt as much, and when Jeff hugs me I don't immediately feel the need to pull away in order to protect it.

I'm working three full days this week instead of only mornings, and this alone gives me an enormous feeling of freedom. I'm no longer tethered to the hospital on a daily basis. My work schedule feels exactly right for me now…the perfect balance between work and rest…between time alone for me to create and write… and time with others.

This afternoon while journaling I suddenly remember the cruise we took last fall, and how I spent a lot of time writing about my deepest wish to be able to work part time at the theatre; to use the days off to pursue my deepening passions for art and writing. I had completely forgotten about this. And now it's like my wish has come true. Of course, I really didn't want to go through breast cancer to get it, but this is the path I was given. This is the road I have traveled.

Wednesday July 10

Today at work I notice how much of my former responsibilities have shifted away from me and onto the shoulders of others. I knew I was giving up projects and tasks when I switched jobs with John, but today I really feel in my body the difference this has made for me. It's strange but utterly delightful to realize I'm no longer the one who has to solve every problem that arises here. I welcome the lighter responsibility as a mountain climber welcomes the removal of a bulky knapsack.

The other day I saw a t-shirt in a catalog that said *I didn't survive breast cancer to die from stress* and I laughed right out loud. That is my new work philosophy in ten words or less!

I tell someone today that I believe my cancer has served its purpose and will not return. She looks at me strangely and as soon as I realize what I've said, I fear that I've spoken too soon, that I will regret these words spoken so bravely out loud. So I temper these thoughts with a wish and a prayer that it will be so. What else is there to do? It is out of my hands; it has always been out of my hands.

Thursday July 11

I'm reading *Full Catastrophe Living* by Jon Kabat-Zinn. The parts about dealing with stress are causing me to look back on the last several years of my life in our stepfamily, to see these years from the perspective that only time allows. Living in the midst of those years I couldn't see the stress that my body, mind and spirit were under. But now I do and I'm stunned at how I allowed it to erode my sense of self; how I surrendered my own bright creative spirit to it.

Kabat-Zinn says that chronic stress lowers the immune system's ability to fight disease. I really think that this contributed in a big way to my cancer. Not that it's anyone's fault really. Certainly not the children's. If anyone is to blame, it's *me* for not caring for myself better. Yet I can't find it in me to be harsh with myself about it. I'm certain that I did the best I could- caring for Jeff, for the kids, and for myself. At this point in my life, the stress is gone and my life has changed. I am once again healthy. I have to view it this way. I have to…or the fear of the cancer returning will create so much stress that my body may lose its defenses again. I will do everything in my power from now on to prevent that from happening.

And then again, I could be wrong. I could have gotten breast cancer because of a fatty diet, lack of exercise, environmental factors, or any one of a number of reasons that scientists are only guessing at now. I will never know, so it's best to make my assumptions and then move on. Better not to dwell on the need for *a reason why*.

The other day I read somewhere online that for most women, breast cancer is just *a blip on the screen of their lives*. A great image. May it be so for me. May it someday be so for all of us.

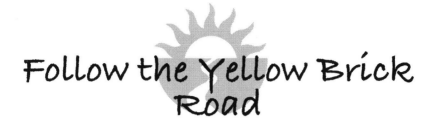

CHAPTER TWENTY-ONE

Follow the Yellow Brick Road

You don't need to be helped any longer.
You've always had the power to go back to Kansas.

— *Glinda to Dorothy in* The Wizard of Oz

Thursday July 18

I walk a mile early this morning and I'm amazed at how good it feels. It's been over three weeks since I've been able to do this. It's 85 degrees and very humid before 7 a.m. but my legs feel strong and I can sense my heart beating in my chest. I'm sweating profusely, but also very much aware of how alive I am. The skin under my radiated breast is almost completely healed, thanks to the ointment Dr. Karp prescribed when he examined me last week. It almost feels like I have my body back again.

The Wizard of Oz opened this week at the theater. Sitting in the audience tonight, I feel as if I've walked directly into the movie. There is Dorothy in her blue gingham dress, carrying Toto tucked under her arm. There's the

Scarecrow who thinks he doesn't have a brain but in reality is the smartest one of them all. There's my friend George playing the silver-suited Tin Man, complaining that he doesn't have a heart when he's really the most loving of them all. And there's the Cowardly Lion who so dearly longs for courage. When I see him trembling with fear, I know exactly how he feels. I know how they all feel. Especially Dorothy, who simply wants to go home. I find myself moved to quiet tears several times during the show. Four characters following the Yellow Brick Road in search of things that seem so out of reach when in reality they already possess them. I see myself in every one of them.

Thursday July 25

Today I'm able to put on a bra for the first time in months. This has a normalizing effect on me. It's been months since I've been able to wear a top without putting a man's shirt on over it! I rummage through my closet for my favorite coral summer sweater and put it on, basking in the bright warmth it brings to my face.

I put Gracie on and glance at myself in the mirror. I stare at myself for a moment, then take the wig off and inspect the small growth of silvery hair that covers my head. It's coming back a little bit wavy and I'm happy about this. It's not even long enough to pass for a short haircut, and yet I no longer look bald. I run my palm over my head. It feels soft and wiry. The beginning of a thought blossoms in my mind. *What if today I leave the wig off?* I'm feeling just brave enough to do it. Solemnly, I place Gracie back on the Styrofoam head in the closet and shut the door.

Giddy with excitement, I email this breaking news to Dawn and she replies right away, encouraging me. She sounds as excited as I feel! When she first stopped wearing her wig, she got a second hole pierced in her ears so she could wear two sets of earrings. It's an excellent idea, one that will make me feel more feminine. I add this to my list of errands for the morning.

As I walk to the car I feel the heat of the sun on my newly liberated scalp. I hold my breath as I walk into the bank, afraid that people will point and stare at me, start whispering about me to their friends. Nothing remotely close to this happens. Everyone acts like practically-bald women come here every day. Well, what do I know? Maybe they do.

At the mall I find a great hat that looks wonderful on me. It's a cap with a little brim, made of several different colored and textured materials. I love it! The young woman at the piercing stand doesn't say anything about my nearly bald head. She goes about the careful business of piercing my ears with the teal studs I have chosen. I admire my new look in the mirror, smiling at myself with tender affection.

Later, I'm looking through some clothes on one of the sales racks at Filene's. An older woman walks right up to me and begins talking. Startled, I look up. She tells me she loves the way I'm wearing my hair! I gulp down the burst of laughter that threatens to escape. She says she really wishes she had the courage to wear her hair so short, then proceeds to say how stunning it looks on me. So... what is the "correct" thing to do, in a situation like this? Do I tell her it's this short because I lost it all to chemo this spring? I start to explain, then stop myself, dreading the look of pity that might be forthcoming. Instead, I simply smile and thank her. This woman has totally made my day. Any doubts I had about ditching the wig have completely flown out the window. When was the last time a stranger came up to me in public and told me they liked my hairstyle?

Driving home, it occurs to me that perhaps the woman is a cancer survivor herself. Perhaps she intuited that my "hairdo" was a result of chemotherapy. Perhaps she remembered her own hair loss, her own first days of going wigless. Perhaps she wanted to mirror my beautiful inner self back to me. I catch my breath in wonder as these thoughts run through my mind. Another layer of joy surrounds my spirit.

When I return from the mall, Merri is in the kitchen making lunch and we chat for a while. I smile in wonder. No one except Jeff has ever seen me without the wig on. I haven't even called him to tell him that I took it off today. The fact that Merri didn't freak out when she saw me like this, the fact that she acts as if this is perfectly normal, is very reassuring.

Friday July 26

It has come to me in the night, this whimsical idea. I was dreaming about being on a journey- a strange and frightening yet wonderful journey. And when I woke up, I clearly saw the parallel between my life and the Oz story. What got those characters down the Yellow Brick Road and home again is exactly what has gotten me through my own journey from diagnosis to recovery: love, courage, and creative intelligence.

Now what I want most of all is a photograph of this new wigless me with the Lion, Scarecrow and Tin Man. This will be a perfect symbol of the journey I've been on. I'll put it in the colorful frame that Dawn sent me earlier this month to celebrate my last radiation treatment. It's bright pink and lime green with a rainbow of polka dots, hearts, stars and flowers around the border. The note with it said: *for a photo of the new and healthy you.* I had put it aside, not quite sure I wanted a photograph taken of me at this stage of the journey, but now I am entirely sure.

I email my friend George (who is playing the Tin Man) to see if he'll ask Casey (Scarecrow) and David (Cowardly Lion) to pose with me on Sunday before or after the matinee. He replies later in the day saying how proud he is of me for taking this next step so soon. He's spoken with the other actors and they're happy and honored to pose with me. I'm filled with a bubbling fizz of excitement, a sparkle that I haven't felt very much this year, and it warms me, moves me forward.

I'm happy that I know myself well enough to know exactly what I need to make ditching this wig a smoother experience. And I'm happy that I love myself enough to ask for what I need, that I'm finding the courage to give myself what I want.

Sunday July 28

I dress carefully for work this morning in my favorite purple skirt and lavender top. I set the patchwork cap on the light gray fuzz that springs from my scalp, and head to the box office. There are five of us working today and no one is shocked to find me wigless. Jeanne, Doug, Dina and Sue all compliment me on my "new look." Part of me wonders if they are just saying this without really meaning it. But after a while, I realize that they are sincere. I may not look front-page-model-beautiful but there has to be a certain glow on my face, simply for summoning up the courage to leave the wig at home. This *is* a new look for me, and I am grateful that my co-workers have noticed, have cared enough to compliment me. I feel so much better about retiring Gracie for good.

During intermission, Sue and I make our way through the crowded lobby, my camera clutched in her hand. We duck behind the big black curtains at the end of the lobby and find George backstage, tall and stiff in his silver Tin Man costume. He introduces me to Casey and the straw in his costume rustles as he gallantly shakes my hand. David hugs me briefly into his soft furry lion suit; he has done many shows here in the past so no introductions are needed.

I stand between David and Casey who put their arms around me, and George leans in beside David. They strike their poses while Sue aims the camera at us and the flash spins in our eyes a few times. Other actors and production staff move noisily around us, drinking water, chatting with friends, busily adjusting sleeves and hemlines.

I thank the three of them as sincerely as I can before Sue and I hurry back to the box office. I wonder if they will ever know how much this means to me.

Thursday August 1

My favorite of the two photos is now in its new frame on my desk. I see a smiling woman clothed in purple, her shorn silvery head sporting a colorful cap and two pairs of earrings. Her body is larger than I remember, but it looks strong and solid, and she is smiling widely, looking directly into the camera. She stands between a very tall bright-faced Scarecrow and a short stubby Lion who is feigning fear. Leaning in next to him is a shy smiling Tin Man clutching his ax. My heart quiets as I study the picture. Yes, this is exactly what I wanted, the perfect symbol of my journey so far this year.

There she stands- the Pilgrim, supported on all sides by Love, Courage, and Intelligence, who have been her companions throughout the entire journey.

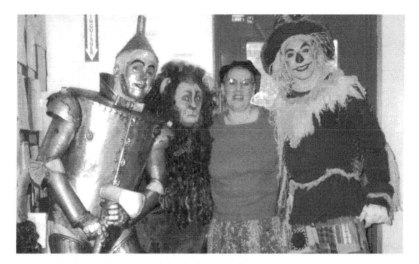

George Dvorsky, David Coffee, Anne Marie Bennett, Casey Colgan, July 2002 at North Shore Music Theatre, Beverly Massachusetts

CHAPTER TWENTY-TWO

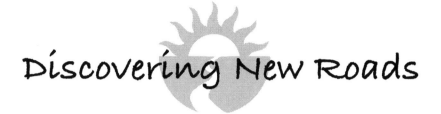

Discovering New Roads

We're fools whether we dance or not,
so we might as well dance.
— Japanese Proverb

Thursday August 29

I've been thinking about the *Weekend for Women Living With Breast Cancer Retreat* that I signed up for in October at Kripalu, a yoga retreat center in the Berkshires. When I got the catalog this spring, I was drawn to it immediately and knew with certainty that I was meant to attend. A weekend with other breast cancer survivors. A weekend just for us. A time to tell our stories, share our strengths, forge a new way forward. And it's being led by Sudha, one of the teachers I remember from my long-ago days at Kripalu. I remember her calm inner strength, her quiet wisdom, her attunement to whoever she was talking with; the way she could always speak the truth with kindness and clarity. It seems that in the intervening years, she has also had breast cancer, three times. I am positive that this weekend will be an expansive experience for me, that it will open me and heal me in ways that I can't imagine right now.

And even though the retreat is for *Women Living With Breast Cancer*, I wonder if I really will fit in. I don't feel like I'm "living with" the cancer anymore. I truly feel that it has left my body. And what I am left with is the Fear of It Coming Back. This is the hardest thing for me now that the treatments are over. Everyone assumes that I've arrived at Normal and am picking up my life where I left off last December. But the reality is completely, utterly different. The reality is this daily fear that I must live with. I find that if I'm consciously breathing and staying in the moment, the fear has much less power to claim me. This is easier said than done, though. It's something that I must practice faithfully every single day.

I'm hoping that the retreat will be able to show me more clearly how to live with the fear. And I'm going to allow the weekend to help me step forward into my own precious future. I'm looking forward to being in the healing environment of Kripalu again… meeting other women on the journey… reaching out my hand and joining them on the road ahead.

Wednesday October 2

We've exchanged our timeshare on Cape Cod for this week in the Berkshires. It's beautiful here. I've been walking every day on the long winding road that borders the mountain. Tonight I soak for a long time in the enormous bathtub. The bubbles are luxurious and exhilarating, the water is hot. Jeff joins me for a while, but it's too warm for him so he gets out and I continue to soak, to read, to relax.

When I finally climb out of the tub an hour later, my body is bright red and it occurs to me that the temperature of the water may have been too hot for my left arm. The thought of possible lymphedema worries me to distraction, and I silently berate myself for not getting out of the tub sooner. I hate having to be so constantly vigilant about my arm.

And yet, as I'm sitting on the bed in my nightgown, rubbing my arm in an attempt to get the lymph fluid moving again, I send a quick word of gratitude to my body for withstanding the physical and emotional stress of this past year, for staying with me and holding strong, in spite of everything.

Thursday October 3

I'm relieved when I get up this morning and see that my arm is fine. I guess I'll be learning to live with the lymphedema-worry as much as I'm learning to live with the fear of the cancer returning.

I'm thinking about my evening prayer ritual, and how I always put the gratitude first. Just this simple practice alone makes me more aware during the course of my day, more aware of these blessings as they're actually happening. Instantaneous gratitude, I guess you'd call it. Being immediately grateful...grateful in each precious moment... noticing... being aware. This has been a major factor in my living with and healing from breast cancer.

Yet I occasionally wonder if what I'm really doing is bargaining with God. Does part of me believe that God will notice my positive attitude, my practice of gratitude, and spare me a recurrence? It scares me every time this thought crosses my mind. Of course, every night I ask that the cancer *not* return. Doesn't everyone? And then I wonder why do I even bother asking for that? Do I really believe in the power of my prayer to stop it from happening? Haven't there been women who prayed and prayed and prayed for it not to return and yet it did? Then why do I think *I* will be any different?

It occurs to me that what I should be praying for instead is the grace to live, to really live, no matter what. Whether the cancer returns or not. This new thought stops me in my tracks. Am I strong enough to pray for this instead?

Thursday October 10

I'm beginning to pack for the weekend, and part of me is already dreading this *Women Living With Breast Cancer* retreat. I know what these Kripalu experiences are like. They are ultimately good for mind, body, and soul. But I'll be expected to open up in order to receive the healing that is ever present there. I know that I will tell my story, and that I will listen to the stories of other women who have walked a similar path these past years. I also know that I will probably cry again, and the thought of this makes me tired. I hear a fearful inner voice urging me to call the reservations line and cancel. It's not too late.

But a deeper part of me will not allow me to do this. I am going to this retreat. There will be no more discussion of it in my mind. I will open myself up to the experience, and I will somehow be transformed. Although I can't imagine being any more inwardly changed than I already am.

Friday October 11

I plop myself onto a comfy chair in front of the largest picture window I can find on the main floor of the Kripalu retreat center, and stare out at the pale gray sky for several minutes. I see distant rain showers falling on the lake and a panorama of mountains laced with autumn-leaved trees. People walk quietly behind me, passing each other in the lobby, speaking softly, laughing, greeting. I'm trying to wind down. Down. Down to the level of least resistance, the level of quiet acceptance. The level of opening.

When was the last time I simply sat and stared out the window like this? The last time I sat in a comfortable chair with nothing to do and nowhere to go? I guess it was during my treatments. Then the treatments stopped and I gradually began to feel better. I got busy again with work, my art and the writing of this book. Now it seems there is no more time for sitting still. Except for right here, right now, this moment.

After dinner, my roommate and I make our way towards one of the smaller program rooms after dinner for the Newcomer's Information Session. There are about 30 people here, sitting on the floor resting against royal blue backjacks. Paula stays out in the hallway to finish her tea as I enter the room. I see a few empty spaces in the front row and go there without hesitation. Hmmm. This is something new already! Ordinarily, I would have taken a seat in the back, attempting to remain anonymous.

The leader of the session introduces himself as Mark. He is tall, handsome and dressed in gray yoga pants and a loose white shirt. He adjusts the microphone, introduces himself, tells a few funny stories to relax us into shared laughter. I turn around to look at the women in the room, trying to discern from the color of their nametags which ones are there for the breast cancer retreat. I see a few and we exchange tentative smiles.

Mark invites us to tell him where we're from and we call out states and countries. There is someone here from England, someone from Canada. The rest of us are from as far away as Seattle, and as close as Springfield. Then he starts calling out the names of the various programs being offered this weekend and invites us to raise our hands when he names the one we're there for. Yoga and Stress. Alive with Yoga. Meditation Retreat. Rest and Renewal. He can't remember any more and asks us to call out the retreats he's forgotten to mention. There is silence.

I hesitate, but only for a second, deciding in that one brief moment that I am proud to be here for this retreat. In another lifetime, I would have looked sadly at someone announcing she was here for a breast cancer retreat. I would have looked at her and thought how awful it must be to go through that; I would have felt glad that it wasn't me. But now *I* am one of *those women*, and I discover that I'm actually glad of it.

Women Living with Breast Cancer, I say loudly and he looks at me with that soft look of pity I've come to expect. I simply smile back at him. He says something nice about Sudha, the retreat leader, and several others raise their hands. I am delighted with myself for speaking up, using my voice, claiming my space. I feel powerful and strong.

 Afterwards, Paula and I make our way to the lower level of the building, turning left and then right in the maze of hallways in the basement. There are already a few women gathered outside of the Lakeview Room, waiting. We introduce ourselves, smiling shyly. One of us is wearing a wig; the rest of us have very short hair, except for Paula who had a different kind of chemo. Her hair is very long and silvery soft. There is an instant companionship that springs up among all of us, an immediate knowing that defies words.

I smile as we enter the room. The lights are soft and low, candles burning everywhere. Someone has hung softly colored silk scarves from the ceiling. There are 18 backjacks arranged in a circle, and in the center is another circle of votive candles which creates the sacred space of an altar.

In the corner there is a slender woman in a flowing lavender top and pants. She is writing with green marker on a large easel pad. This is Sudha, an older Sudha than I remember. But then I'm older too, I remind myself. I realize with a shock that her beautiful long "Breck Girl" tresses are gone and in their place is hair that's a bit thinner and longer than mine. I realize that I was expecting her to look the same as she did twelve years ago when I last saw her here. But of course, she's lost her hair too. How silly of me to not think of this.

She writes quickly and with large strokes WOMEN LIVING WITH BREAST CANCER, then underlines the word LIVING several times. She pauses for a moment and turns around, letting her friendly gaze sweep around the gathering circle of women. Some of us are leaning against the backjacks, some are already quietly chatting with each other. She smiles when I meet her eyes, and there is a light within her that is clear and strong. Yes, this is the same Sudha. This is the one I remember.

She tells us about the weekend's agenda, introduces us to her four program assistants, and talks a little about what life at Kripalu is like. Then she says we'll take turns introducing ourselves and placing the item we brought from home in the circular altar ringed with white candles.

The item we brought from home. I suddenly remember that we were supposed to bring something precious to us, something that symbolizes joy. I have completely forgotten this. It must be my new and unimproved "chemo brain" because I used to be the kind of person who would never forget something like this. My mind scrambles frantically for something to place on the altar and I look in my tote bag for clues. I see my journal, a sweater, a pen, and the book I was reading before I met Paula for supper. It's called *Spiritual Journeys Along the Yellow Brick Road* by Darren John Main.

One by one we place on the altar those things that are most meaningful for us. A journal. A family portrait. A necklace of precious stones that was a special gift. A candle. A bracelet. A statue of a woman, her arms raised in victory. A rock from a prayer garden.

As each woman lays her object down, she introduces herself, gives a tiny bit of her background, sharing how she has come to be here today. Some women, like me, are finished with treatments. Some are just beginning. Some are halfway through. A few women have had recurrences. One woman says that she has been cancer-free for 32 years and tears spring to my eyes immediately. A big sigh of hope goes around the circle.

When it's my turn, I lay the book on the altar and I speak of the photo of myself with the Scarecrow, Tin Man, and Lion. I talk about the symbolism this has for me and I notice others who are nodding in affirmation. Their validation massages my spirit with a wonderful calm joy.

All of our precious objects remain in the center of the circle. Throughout the weekend they are to be a reminder of who we are, a constant naming to us of all that is sacred, precious, sweet.

Saturday October 12

This morning we divide into groups of three and take turns telling our stories. I sit in a small circle, knee-to-knee with Kathleen and Barbara, both of whom have the most beautiful smiles, the most radiant spirits. In the past I would have volunteered to go first in order to get it over with. Today I volunteer because I'm excited to be telling my story in the presence of women who will understand. I want to go first because I'm eager to speak the truth of my journey in such a sacred space.

So I do go first, and parts of my story are accompanied by tears. But they are not the tears of painful memories. I'm crying because the emotions connected with my recent journey are still so tender, and because the spiritual generosity of these women who are listening, *really listening* to me, is so utterly validating that it sets my heart free.

Barbara and Kathleen each tell their stories also, and I listen to them with a full heart and reverent ear. The minute details of our individual journeys are so different (a lumpectomy, a double mastectomy, different kinds of chemo), yet the underlying feelings are the same.

The rest of the weekend is full of true camaraderie, a blossoming of friendship among women who have walked and are walking the path together, not alone as some of us have imagined.

We walk a beautiful seven-circuit labyrinth in the middle of a meadow surrounded by autumn-shaded flowers and trees, and I learn a visceral lesson in Trust that surprises and delights me. I'm able to trust that each step is leading me closer to the center, even though it's hard to see this as I slowly put one foot in front of the other on the path.

We dance together in an hour of soul-shaking Kripalu DansKinetics®, and I'm filled with the immediate, forgotten knowledge that my body is sacred, that moving like this places me directly in touch with the child inside me who longs to run and dance and play.

We practice gentle yoga together, and I begin to let go of the fear that I will hurt my surgical arm.

We sing together and I cherish the words. *Return to what you are, return to who you are, return to where you are, born and reborn again.*

We breathe deeply together and the silence is passed around the circle like golden orbs of peace that settle deeply into our bodies and souls.

We discuss things that have helped us on our journey and we talk about the fear of recurrence. We talk about how the cancer has changed our perceptions of ourselves, how it has changed the way we experience sexuality, how it has transformed our bodies, our minds, our spirits.

We cry together, and we laugh together. Our sorrows are softened, changed, healed.

Sunday October 13

On our last evening together, we meet in the women's locker room to get ready for an hour in the hot tub. We take off all our clothes and make a sweet ritual of adorning our bodies with temporary tattoos. I place a rose tattoo on my left breast, and a smaller one right above the node dissection scar, which is long and pink and shiny now, still tender to the touch. I smile, imagining Dr. Karp's surprise next week when he examines me.

We lower ourselves into the big tub of hot frothy bubbles- singing, laughing, shouting to one another above the roar of the water. Women surround me. All of us are stark naked. We have bodies and scars of varying size, shape, and hue. Women's bodies, one and all, scarred but unmistakably beautiful.

Each face glows with an inner strength that defies the presence of the scars... defies and transforms them into sacred markings that are to be praised, worshipped, and most definitely loved. All kinds of bodies- tall, short, light, dark, thin, heavy, lumpy, slender, smooth, marked, unmarked, breasts, no breasts, reconstructions in all stages, node dissection scars, tram flap scars, mastectomy scars. There are women here who can't bear to get undressed in front of their partners. Women who act like they bathe naked with friends every night. Women who have never shown another living soul their cancer-carved bodies.

I look around me, sweating in the humid steam rising from the water, and I feel privileged to be standing here in the company of these women. Privileged. Honored. Special. Chosen.

I am one of them. I'm not just observing. I too bear the scars of two lumpectomies and a full node dissection. I am one of them. This knowledge awes and humbles me. I am one of the women now *living* with breast cancer and all that that implies. Even though I still have my breasts, and even though my scars are not as large, vivid, or painful as some. I am one of them, and I am glad.

After the whirlpool, we dress and gather in the program room for Shamanic dance. We are given blindfolds and encouraged to wear them although it's not mandatory. Sudha encourages us to sit still on the floor for a while and just listen to the music, allow it to penetrate our bodies, then move with and to the music however our bodies want to move. I put on the blindfold and wait as the music begins. Sudha tells us that she and the four program assistants will be holding space for us, keeping us from hurting ourselves, keeping us from crashing into each other and into the walls. It's a little hard to imagine this since it's not that big of a room and there are four concrete poles spaced throughout the center of it, but I choose to trust.

I choose to let go of my preconceived definitions of myself. I choose to let my body, heavy as it is, move as it will. I choose to stop thinking about time, about how I look. I choose to be in this present moment, with the music, my body, and the dance.

Sudha demonstrates a Shamanic breath (in, in, out) and encourages us to keep that rhythm in our breathing throughout the dance. At first I simply stand still and sway to the music in my own small space on the floor. Listening. Feeling.

A few times I hear Sudha call out over the drumming, throbbing beat of the music, *Dance this dance for yourself. Dance the dance of your life.* I take these words into my being and translate them into my dance. I give in to the driving beat of the music and start to dance, allowing myself to trust this blossoming energy in my body. There is sacred pleasure in this trust. I find a joyful thrumming bliss in the movement of my body.

I am dancing a dance of gratitude for my life, for all of the people who have traveled with me on my journey. Soon I am leaping, twirling, spinning. The freedom I'm experiencing is deeply exhilarating. Many times I feel gentle hands on my back, my shoulders, facing me in another direction, and I simply allow myself to be turned. The redirection becomes part of the dance.

When the music slows down and quietly fades away, we lay on our backs on the floor. Soft, sweet music flows around our perspiring bodies.

The word *Alleluia* is being sung over and over and over again. It sounds like angels singing. Perhaps it is.

Sudha and her assistants come to each of us. When they join me, they sit on the floor around me and lay hands on my head, my arms, my legs, my feet. I'm crying quietly now, tears of joy and healing, tears of release and self-acceptance.

I hear Sudha's gentle voice telling me to breathe through my mouth, to not hold back, to continue to allow the tears. So I let the warm tears slide down my cheeks and into my ears. I feel so loved, so lifted, so immense, so whole, so real.

Keep breathing, her voice says softly, and I do exactly that.

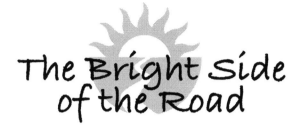

The Bright Side
of the Road

Although no one can go back and make a brand new start,
anyone can start now and make a brand new ending.
— Carl Bard

This story has been about a single journey within the bigger, broader journey of my life.

Thank you, dear reader, for coming along with me on this journey. I have relived it over and over through successive writings and re-writings of this manuscript. Each time I've relived it, I've been aware of your presence, and grateful that you have taken the time to accompany me on my journey.

Today as I write this, it has been almost seven years since my breast cancer treatments ended. And yet, my journey continues...

Several times in the last seven years, I have looked at the path before me and thought it impossible to go on as it seemed so rocky, so steep. I was demoted unfairly at the theatre where I worked, and chose to leave. Jeff was diagnosed with prostate cancer, and survived. My mother had a stroke and died several days later (the night before Jeff's surgery). Our beloved tiger cat, Scooter, disappeared and never came back. I've had a few scares with iffy mammograms.

But also during the last seven years, there have been long periods of smooth sailing, where I skip along on the smooth and even path as if I were five years old, carefree and content. My hair grew back (still curly, hooray!), I found a therapist, I began exercising, I found a true and powerful art process called SoulCollage® and took the training to become a Facilitator. Jeff and I now have five grandchildren (with one more on the way). I am spending my days writing, creating art, facilitating SoulCollage® in person and online, and building my business, KaleidoSoul.

I write this as a reminder that we are all on journeys, individual yet connected.

Sometimes the road I'm on will be rocky and difficult; sometimes it will be smooth and easy. But I always move forward with my now clear understanding that I can *choose* the dark side or the bright side of the road.

I choose the bright side.

It doesn't lessen the height of any mountain I face, nor does it smooth out the jagged potholes that cause me to stumble. What walking on the bright side does is illuminate the path I am on so that my inner vision is clearer.

The important thing to remember is this: the choice is always mine.

Touchstones for Body, Mind and Spirit

A Journey with Breast Cancer is not a separate journey with a distinct beginning, middle, and end. Everyone gifted with this diagnosis embarks on the journey already equipped with resources that their life has provided for them. During the experience with cancer and after the treatments are over, these resources become even more valuable travel gear.

For me, these resources were (and continue to be): visualization, affirmations, yoga, meditation, solitude, art, books, music, theatre, journaling, connection to a power greater than myself, and connection to others.

I share the following suggestions with you in the hope that, no matter where you are on this journey, you will be able to choose and name touchstones for yourself so that your path will steer you towards your own bright side of the road. Your touchstones may be the same; they may be different. Please take what you like and leave the rest.

Feel your feelings. Don't push them away. Find a way to acknowledge your feelings to yourself. Find a way to express your feelings so they don't stay locked inside of you: write them in a notebook, fling them out with crayons or paint, dance with them, tell them to a trusted friend.

Notice what you are grateful for. Make gratitude lists, either in your journal or in a computer document, or just in your heart at the end of every day. Revisit your lists often for encouragement and inspiration.

Stay present with yourself. It is so tempting to push aside the difficult feelings, but it's more important to feel them as they arise. They don't last forever. But they do go underground and cause more pain if you ignore them.

Slow down your life as much as you can so you can remain connected to yourself.

Remain as much as you can in the present moment. This is the only moment you have. Right now, right here.

Ask others to pray for you. If you don't believe in prayer, ask them to send positive, loving thoughts your way.

Ask for help when you need it. Family, friends and others may be waiting in the wings looking for direction from you so they can show you how much they love and care for you.

Use or adapt the simple prayer: *God, you are here. God, I am here.*

Seek things that will make you laugh: watch a funny TV show, rent a silly movie, read a witty book, play with a baby. Remember, you know yourself best. What is it that makes *you* laugh?

Remember, when deciding who to tell or not tell about your diagnosis, *you* are the one who is in charge. *You* get to decide who knows and who doesn't know. Choose to tell people who respect and love you; choose to tell people in whose presence you feel safe.

Focus on *yourself* when you are telling people about your diagnosis. It doesn't matter how they are "taking" it. You are not responsible for making them feel better about what is happening to *you*.

Draw boundaries wherever you need them. It's perfectly okay to say "no" to something that someone offers you. You can do so with kindness and gratitude.

Use affirmations daily. Create your own or use the ones listed in Appendix Two.

Whine and complain. It's totally okay. Living a journey into the "bright side of the road" doesn't mean that you act cheerful all the time. What really matters is your own self-acceptance and inner honesty.

Create an altar (small or large), which is a sacred space that will remind you of your beautiful soul and of this larger journey you are on. Choose objects that comfort and inspire you. Choose things that visually express Spirit to you in some way.

Be aware of the choices you are making on a daily basis. I'm talking about the decisions you make as far as surgeries and treatments are concerned, as well as the bigger choices of your journey: gratitude or depression, community or isolation, bright side or dark side, feelings or numbness, rest or work. Remember that the choices you make give you power and control over your life during this strange and unexpected journey. And the choices you make should be *yours*, based on what *you* need and want, not based on what *others* think you should be doing.

Be kind to your inner child during the steep parts of the journey. What comforts her the most? Mine loves bubble baths, teddy bears and reading good novels, so I indulged her in these as often as I could. Take a quiet moment and ask your inner child what she would like to do right now, and really listen for her answer. Then do what she suggests if you possibly can.

Choose a talisman that is small enough to carry with you to your appointments, or to hold onto when you are feeling low. Choose something that has special meaning for you. As soon as you see it or touch it, it should put you in touch with your soul, with your relationship with Spirit.

Connect to others in whatever way feels most comfortable and safe to you. This might mean emails and online groups, or it might mean in-person support groups or nights out with friends. You are not alone on this journey. Find a way to reinforce that for yourself.

Pamper your body in whatever way feels good to you. Get a massage, treat yourself to a pedicure, take a warm bath, slide into a nap, buy a luxuriously soft sweater that feels good against your skin, take a short walk in the sunshine.

Ask yourself repeatedly: What do I need? How can I give myself what I need?

Listen to your night dreams. Write about them in your journal. Ask yourself what they might mean.

Honor and respect your daydreams. Write about them in your journal. Ask yourself how you can make them come true.

Create a short daily ritual that lifts and sustains you. Ritual is a repeated activity that connects us with the Divine. Every night before sleep rolled in, I shut my eyes and listed what I was grateful for, asked for what I needed and then said a few prayers for others. This was short and simple, yet very powerful.

Create or participate in a ritual that is more elaborate and formal. You might attend a daily Mass, recite prayers from your religion's Prayer Book, light a candle and stare into the flame, meditate on a certain word or scripture, take a walk, write a daily prayer in your journal... or whatever speaks to *your* soul. It doesn't have to be done at the same time every day. And if you skip a day (accidentally or on purpose), please don't beat yourself up. This is meant to lift and sustain you. It is not another reason to be hard on yourself.

Whisper "I love you" to your face in the mirror every morning. Or shout it!

Practice forgiveness, of yourself and others. Are there people in your past that you need to forgive? Do you need to forgive *yourself*? This is a book that I found especially helpful when working with forgiveness: *The Art of Forgiveness, Lovingkindness and Peace*, by Jack Kornfield.

Give yourself something to look forward to. This could be as simple as inviting a friend over to play cards, or as involved as planning a special trip once your treatments are over. What would please *you* most?

Write down absolutely everything you are thinking and feeling into a letter or journal and share it with someone you love, or write it in your journal and don't show a soul. Let the feelings and thoughts come up naturally. And *feel* them as you write them. Expression... getting it all out of your body... that's the most important thing.

Affirmations That Helped Me on My Journey

An affirmation is a positive statement designed to counteract a negative belief that you have about yourself or about something in your environment. It should be written in the present tense and should re-affirm something that you want to become true.

By using an affirmation, you are attempting to convince yourself that you can do or be something even though your mind doesn't accept it yet. I found that affirmations worked best when I said them out loud to myself, several times in a row, several times a day. You can also record them and listen to yourself saying them over and over. Another thing I found helpful with my affirmation work was writing them on little note cards or sticky notes and placing them in strategic locations where I would see them often: the bathroom mirror, the fridge, my nightstand, the computer monitor…etc. In using affirmations on your breast cancer journey, you are re-programming your mind away from negativity and towards brightness. I have found that this is one of the most healing tools I possessed, both on that journey as well as afterwards. Below are the ones that helped me the most, but this list is by no means conclusive. Feel free to use any affirmations here that you are drawn to. The affirmations themselves are not copyrighted.

Also, feel free to use any affirmations here as stepping-stones to creating your own. Using your own words is always a good way to start.

❄ I am glad to be alive.

❄ Just for today, I am healthy.

❄ All is well.

❄ I am beautiful just as I am.

❄ I face my fears with courage and they turn to love.

❄ I am filled with healing white light.

❄ My immune system is fully functioning, healthy, and strong.

❄ I am safe.

❄ My body is healthy and strong.

❄ Hands larger than mine are guiding me through this and every journey.

❄ I am well-loved. I am surrounded by people who love and care for me.

❄ I am finding my way to what is next.

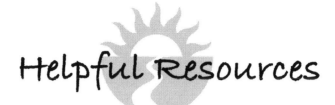

Helpful Resources

This section holds information on the books, articles, topics, websites and other resources that I mentioned throughout my story. It also contains resources that have helped me stay on the bright side of the road since my treatments ended.

Your resources may be the same; they may be different. Please take what you like and leave the rest.

Books About Cancer:

Affirmations, Meditations and Encouragements for Women Living with Breast Cancer, by Linda Dackman. 1993. Harpercollins.

Guided by Dreams: Breast Cancer, Dreams, and Transformation, by Rachel Norment. 2006. Brandylane.

Spinning Straw Into Gold: Your Emotional Recovery From Breast Cancer, by Ronnie Kaye. 1991. Fireside.

Surviving Cancer, by Margie Levine. 2001. Broadway Books.

Books that Lifted My Spirit and Made Me Smile

All I Want Is a Warm Bed and a Kind Word and Unlimited Power, by Ashleigh Brilliant. 1985. Woodbridge Press.

Everything Here Is Mine: An Unhelpful Guide to Cat Behavior, by Nicole Hollander. 2000. Sourcebooks Hysteria.

The Blue Day Book, by Bradley Trevor Greive. 2000. Andrews McMeel.

The Indispensable Calvin And Hobbes, by Bill Watterson. 1992. Andrews McMeel.

Books About the Mind-Body Connection

Anatomy of an Illness as Perceived by the Patient: Reflections on Healing and Regeneration, by Norman Cousins. 2001. W. W. Norton & Company.

Full Catastrophe Living: Using the Wisdom of Your Body and Mind to Face Stress, Pain, and Illness, by Jon Kabat-Zinn. 1990. Delta.

Love, Medicine and Miracles: Lessons Learned about Self-Healing from a Surgeon's Experience with Exceptional Patients, by Bernie S. Siegel. 1990. Harper Paperbacks.

Peace, Love and Healing: Bodymind Communication & the Path to Self-Healing: An Exploration, by Bernie S. Siegel. 1990. Harper Paperbacks.

The Art of Forgiveness, Lovingkindness and Peace, by Jack Kornfield. 2002. Bantam.

Books About Affirmations:

Create Your Own Affirmations: A Creative Visualization Kit, by Shakti Gawain. 2003. New World Library.

Meditations to Heal Your Life, by Louise Hay. 2002. Hay House.

Books About Journeys:

Every Good and Perfect Gift, by Brenda Jernigan. 2001. Harmony.

Learning to Fall: The Blessings of an Imperfect Life, by Philip Simmons. 2002. Bantam.

Spiritual Journeys Along the Yellow Brick Road, by Darren John Main. 2000. Findhorn Press.

Books About Art and Healing:

Art Heals: How Creativity Cures the Soul, by Shaun McNiff. 2004. Shambhala.

SoulCollage: An Intuitive Collage Process for Individuals and Groups, by Seena B. Frost. 2001, revised 2009. Hanford Mead.

The Art of Emotional Healing, by Lucia Capacchione. 2006. Shambhala.

The Soul's Palette: Drawing on Art's Transformative Powers, by Cathy A. Malchiodi. 2002. Shambhala.

Books About Guided Imagery/Visualization:

Creative Meditation and Visualization, by David Fontana. 2007. Watkins.

Guided Imagery for Self-Healing, by Martin Rossman. 2000. HJ Kramer/ New World Library.

Imagery in You: Mining for Treasure in Your Inner World, by Jenny Garrison. 2006. Outskirts Press.

The Joy of Visualization, by Valerie Wells. 1990. Chronicle Books.

Books About Living a Full and Joyful Life:

Slow Time: Recovering the Natural Rhythm of Life, by Waverly Fitzgerald. 2008. Priestess of Swords Press.

The Pathway: Follow the Road to Health and Happiness, by Laurel Mellin. 2003. Collins Living.

Woman's Retreat Book: A Guide to Restoring, Rediscovering and Reawakening Your True Self — In a Moment, An Hour, Or a Weekend, by Jennifer Louden. 2005. HarperOne.

Online:

Artella Words and Art: This site feeds my need for verbal and artistic expression. *www.artellawordsandart.com*

Breast Cancer Survivor's Online Group: This is the group that helped me the most during my journey. And it's where I met Dawn and Elizabeth! *www.bcsupport.org*

Breast Cancer Stories: This is an excellent site where you can search for survivors' stories by location, age, and/or type of breast cancer. You can also submit your own story and share with others. *www.breastcancerstories.org*

Comfort Café: This is Jennifer Louden's absolutely amazing site where women go for sweet dollops of self-care and self-kindness. An important tool for any woman, breast cancer or not. *www.comfortqueen.com/comfortcafe*

KaleidoSoul: *Spinning the Fragments of Your World Into Wholeness and Beauty Through SoulCollage®.* This is my website which is dedicated to the art and practice of SoulCollage® as created by Seena Frost. SoulCollage® is a powerful tool that helped me (and is helping me) integrate my breast cancer experience into my life's journey in a visual, creative way using very simple materials (magazine images, scissors and glue).
www.kaleidosoul.com/breastcancer.html

The Solution Method- This site expands and offers community for those who are following Laurel Mellin's book, *The Pathway* (see above). The focus here is on rewiring our brains from stress to joy. This method helps me to keep my emotions in balance, as well as to stay deeply connected to myself. *www.solutionmethod.org*

Movies/TV:

Vicar of Dibley (TV series), featuring Dawn French. BBC Video.

Wit, featuring Emma Thompson. HBO Pictures. 2001.

Wizard of Oz, featuring Judy Garland, Ray Bolger, Bert Lahr. 1939.

Audio:

Creative Visualization Meditations, by Shakti Gawain and Marc Allen. 2002. New World Library.

Health Journeys – Has an excellent series of guided meditations that are specifically for preparing for surgery, and going through cancer treatments. They can all be purchased as cassettes, CD's or downloaded as mp3 files. *www.healthjourneys.com*

Magical Inner Journey - Circle of Community - This is the guided meditation that I created for relaxation before my surgeries. If you like, you can download it as an mp3 file on this page: *www.annemariebennett.com/brightside.html*

Ragtime - The Musical, featuring Brian Stokes Mitchell and Audra McDonald.

Whispers of Spirit & Happiness: Affirmational Soundtracks for Positive Learning, by Deepak Chopra and Don Miguel Ruiz. 2008. The Relaxation Company.

Magazines:

How to Pray, magazine article by Lindsey Crittenden. Published by *Real Simple Magazine.* November-December 2001.

Oprah Magazine - *www.oprah.com*

Other:

Soft Head Scarves - These come in a huge variety of colors and patterns. Absolutely beautiful! *www.4women.com*

Places:

Lahey Clinic - This is the hospital where I was treated. Note that Dr. Morganstern is no longer at Lahey, but has transferred to Dana-Farber Hospital in Boston. *www.lahey.org*

Kripalu Center for Yoga and Health - A retreat center offering get-aways on all manner of things that have to do with body, mind and spirit. Located in Lenox, Massachusetts. *www.kripalu.org*

The Healing Garden - A non-profit organization that provides counseling and complementary therapies for women with breast cancer. Located in Harvard, Massachusetts. *www.healinggarden.net*

Please feel free to share with me any resources that helped/are helping you on your own "bright side of the road" journey:
annemarie@annemariebennett.com

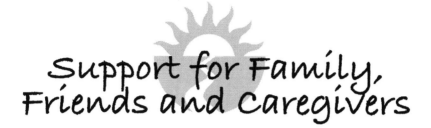

Support for Family, Friends and Caregivers

Here is a list of things that were helpful in terms of how others responded to me during my breast cancer journey. Again, what works for one person might not work for another. Please take what you like and leave the rest.

Don'ts

Don't say "you look great" when you know she doesn't. It's really not necessary to comment on her appearance.

Don't just say "Let me know if there's something I can do." Instead try offering specific modes of help: "How would it be if I come over on Friday and clean your kitchen for you?" or "I'm making a chicken casserole for my family this afternoon. Would you like it if I doubled the recipe and brought you dinner tonight?"

Don't stare at her chest.

Don't make assumptions. This is her journey, not yours. You might love chatting about your experience 'til the cows come home, but she might be more reserved and quiet. Don't expect her to respond or react the way you would.

Don't feel sorry for her. Empathy is a whole different thing from pity.

Don't be afraid of disturbing her. If she doesn't feel like talking or answering the phone, she will let it go to voicemail. Leave her a message. Send her an email and invite her to call you when she feels up to it.

Do's

Do keep *yourself* on your *own* bright side of the road. There's no way you can be a support to someone going through breast cancer if you aren't present for yourself first.

Do send a card and/or a "real" letter in the mail every once in a while. Email is all well and good, but there's nothing like getting something in the mail that is addressed to you and you alone.

Do offer: premade meals, babysitting, cleaning, rides to appointments, an afternoon at the movies, a massage, a pedicure... or something else that she needs or wants.

Do ask questions about what she is going through. These can be specific, about her physical symptoms, about her surgery, whether or not she likes her doctors. If you sense that she would like to talk more but doesn't know how, don't be satisfied with one or two word answers. Ask more detailed questions to help her express the experience.

Do ask more general questions as well, such as Dr. Morganstern's "How is your spirit?"

Do listen inside yourself and discern what *you* are particularly curious about. If she had just returned from a trip to somewhere you'd never been, you'd be curious about the details, right? This is pretty much the same thing: she's on a journey that you can't go on with her. Ask her what you want to know.

Do send or bring flowers. Take the time to find out what her favorite flowers actually are. Don't send her what *you* would like. Send her something that you know *she* likes.

Do send her something funny that will make her laugh. The importance of laugher cannot be underestimated here.

Do say "I love you." Say "I'll help you get through this" or "We'll get through this together." Words are very powerful. Words make a big difference. Words matter.

Do stay in the moment when you are with her. Pay close attention to your *own* feelings. Give *yourself* love and encouragement. Remind yourself that whatever *you* are feeling is perfectly acceptable and okay.

Do create your own affirmations (see Appendix Two) to help you through this. It's not easy to watch someone you love go through breast cancer treatments.

Do treat her like "normal." Tell her about what's going on with you. Keep her up to date on what is happening with family and friends.

Do affirm her feelings, even if they are not "pretty" or "clear." You can mirror them back to her so that she feels heard and seen ("What I hear you saying is..."). You don't have to take responsibility for her feelings, nor do you have to make them go away.

Do look at her. Slow down and really *see* her. Ask her about her hobbies (even if they are on the back burner for now), interests, pets, children, what books she is reading, if there's anything in the future she is looking forward to.

Do remember that when her treatments are over, the journey continues. Continue to follow the above do's and don'ts which will remind her that you are there for her even though her appointments and medications have stopped.

If you are a family member, friend, or caregiver to someone on a breast cancer journey, please feel free to share any additional suggestions and/or resources that you find helpful: annemarie@annemariebennett.com

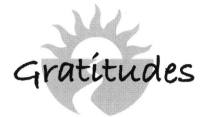

Gratitudes

First of all, I never intended to write a book. During my diagnosis, surgeries and treatments, my journal entries were simply journal entries. I have kept a journal since I was 16 years old, and I write to express whatever I am feeling and going through on a continual basis.

After the weekend at Kripalu in October of 2002, I re-read my journals from the time right before my diagnosis until the end of the retreat. Looking at the "big picture" of my journey, I felt a huge inner prompting to share my journey with other women who were going through the same thing.

I still wasn't intending to write a book. A magazine article was forming in my mind, based on these journal entries. So I started typing what I'd written in my journals into my laptop, entry by entry. This is how the book came to be: the story just wouldn't fit itself into a short article!

The process of writing *Bright Side of the Road* has turned into a journey in and of itself. Along the way of both journeys, I have learned about the power of gratitude. So I use this space here to give voice to how grateful I am to the following members of my Community:

Thank you to my team at Lahey Clinic in Peabody and Burlington, Massachusetts, especially Dr. Stephen Karp, Dr. Daniel Morganstern, and Dr. Lyubov Girshovich. The Tender Loving Care I received on this journey from the entire staff at Lahey made a world of difference in my healing.

Thank you to George Dvorsky, David Coffee, and Casey Colgan, for permission to use your photo in Chapter 21. Your generosity of spirit in agreeing to pose with me in 2002, and in agreeing to let me use the photo now, is so appreciated.

Thank you to Dawn and Elizabeth. I truly do bless the day I found you both on the Breast Cancer Survivor's Board. Your presence on my journey brought me so much hope and comfort when I discovered I wasn't alone.

Thank you to my brother Joe, for reading several drafts of this book with a fine tooth comb (and red pen!). The insight and wisdom you brought to my editing process has been invaluable. And your encouragement and thoughtfulness during my surgeries and treatments made the journey so much easier to navigate.

Thank you to my niece Stephanie, for your love and support throughout my journey… and for spending an entire afternoon shooting photos of me for the back cover. You make me look so beautiful!

Thank you to my family for all your love and prayers along the way: Joe, Karen, Allison, Stephanie, John, Maryann, Mike and Pete.

Thank you to Mom and Dad, who always encouraged my writing. I know that you are still with us in Spirit. I thank you both for the love that framed my birth.

Thank you to Joanna Powell Colbert for designing this book with grace and style. I completely trusted you with my manuscript and you took it into your heart and made it as beautiful as I imagined it would be.

Thank you to those from our worldwide SoulCollage® Community who so graciously volunteered to read the manuscript and gave me such heartfelt responses and suggestions: Elaine Vallante in Massachusetts, Marti Beddoe in Illinois, Lisa Plummer in Virginia, Claire Gillen in the U.K., Dot Fielder in Tennessee, and Stacey Apeitos in Australia. I welcomed each and every one of your comments and suggestions, which helped me to put the finishing touches on the final draft.

Thank you to Elaine Vallante. I treasure our friendship. I wish I'd known you when I was going through my cancer journey; you are everything that a person needs in a friend, and more. You have been there for me every step of the way these past five years. Your encouragement and support as I've been writing this book mean the world to me.

Thank you to Cheryl Finley, a "soul sister" in the deepest sense of that phrase. I am so happy that we found each other through KaleidoSoul! Sharing our journeys together has been one of the highlights of my life these last few years.

Thank you to Fran Booth, who walked with me on the journey of healing for four years after my treatments were over. You gave me space to listen inside; you gave me permission to feel and embrace everything. I wish that everyone on this journey could have someone like you on their side!

Thank you to Sudha (Carolyn Lundeen). Your *Retreat for Women Living with Breast Cancer* weekend that I attended at Kripalu was an amazing gift, a healing adventure, and a turning point on my journey. I am grateful to you for stepping forward and sharing your experience, hope and strength with us in such a loving, creative way.

Thank you to Seena Frost, creator of the intuitive art process SoulCollage® which has touched my life in such a huge way. I wish I'd known about SoulCollage® when I was going through my breast cancer journey because it would have made the journey even brighter for me. Thank you for this simple yet deep gift you have given to the world.

Thank you to Sasha, Scooter and Minnie. I know you'll never read this book or be happy to see your name in print in this section, but I need to put it here for the world to see. There is power and healing in the love of a good pet, and the three of you have blessed me a million times with your presence.

Thank you to Amanda, Jeffrey, and Merri. I am happy to be your stepmother. I appreciate the loving ways that you touched my life during my treatments. And thank you for all these beautiful grandchildren who grace our lives with laughter and joy: Jordan, Jason, Tori, Lissy, Camden (and he/she-who-is-yet-to-be-named)!

And finally, thank you to Jeff. I feel extraordinarily blessed to be married to you. You are my love, my strength, my home. When I was first diagnosed, your immediate response was "We'll get through this together." And you saw to it that we did. Thank you with all my heart for loving me no matter what, and for accepting me, warts and all. I could not ask for a sweeter, gentler, more compassionate companion for this journey.

And all shall be well,
and all shall be well,
and all manner of thing
shall be well.

— Julian of Norwich

3676074

Made in the USA